BODY MEASUREMENTS TRACKER

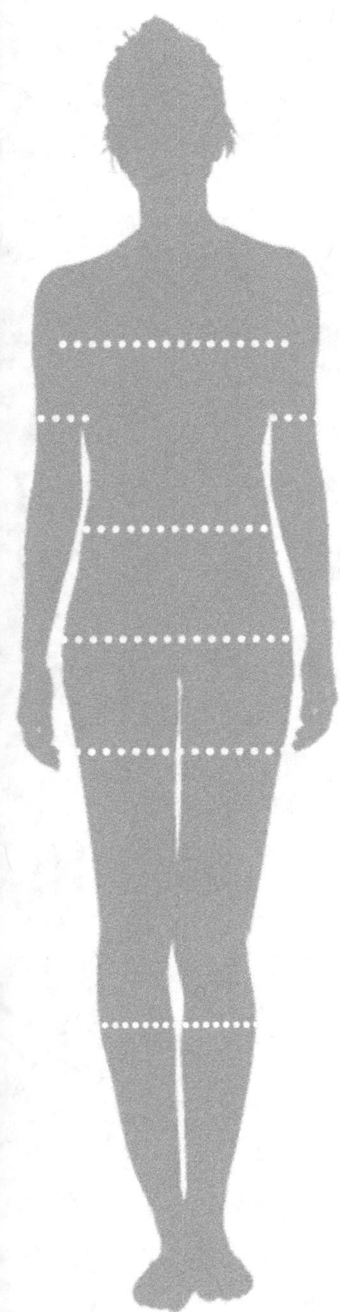

	BEFORE	AFTER
DATE		
CHEST		
LEFT ARM		LEFT ARM
RIGHT ARM		RIGHT ARM
WAIST		WAIST
HIPS		HIPS
LEFT THIGH		LEFT THIGH
RIGHT THIGH		RIGHT THIGH
LEFT CALF		LEFT CALF
RIGHT CALF		RIGHT CALF
WEIGHT		WEIGHT
NOTES		

BODY MEASUREMENTS TRACKER

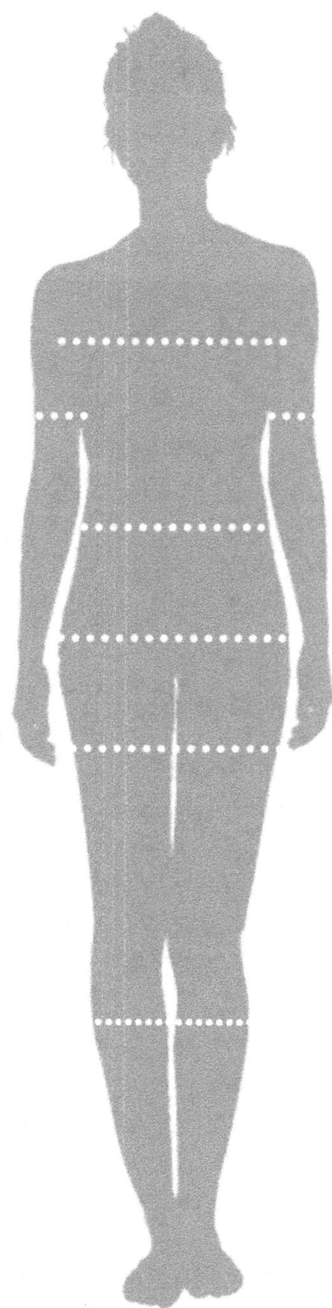

	BEFORE	AFTER
DATE		
CHEST		
LEFT ARM		
RIGHT ARM		
WAIST		
HIPS		
LEFT THIGH		
RIGHT THIGH		
LEFT CALF		
RIGHT CALF		
WEIGHT		
NOTES		

BODY MEASUREMENTS TRACKER

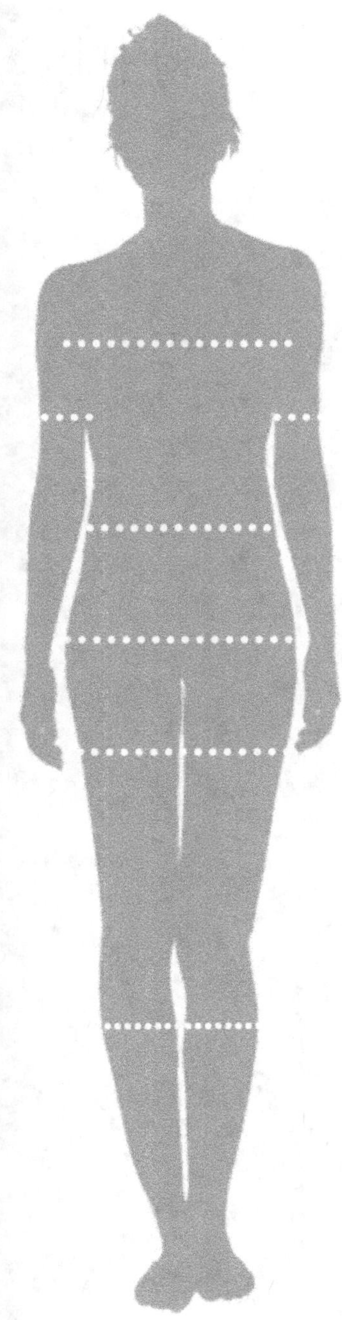

	BEFORE	AFTER
DATE		
CHEST		
LEFT ARM		
RIGHT ARM		
WAIST		
HIPS		
LEFT THIGH		
RIGHT THIGH		
LEFT CALF		
RIGHT CALF		
WEIGHT		
NOTES		

BODY MEASUREMENTS TRACKER

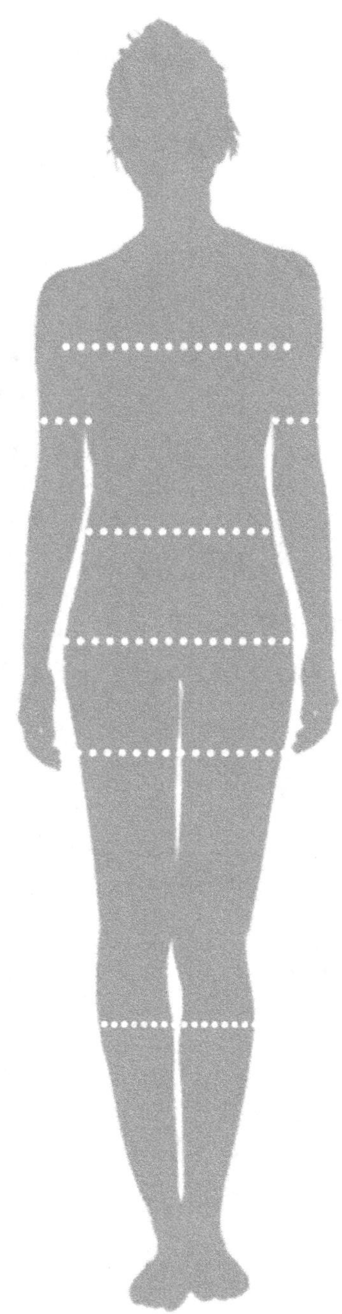

BEFORE

DATE

CHEST

LEFT ARM

RIGHT ARM

WAIST

HIPS

LEFT THIGH

RIGHT THIGH

LEFT CALF

RIGHT CALF

WEIGHT

NOTES

AFTER

DATE

CHEST

LEFT ARM

RIGHT ARM

WAIST

HIPS

LEFT THIGH

RIGHT THIGH

LEFT CALF

RIGHT CALF

WEIGHT

BODY MEASUREMENTS TRACKER

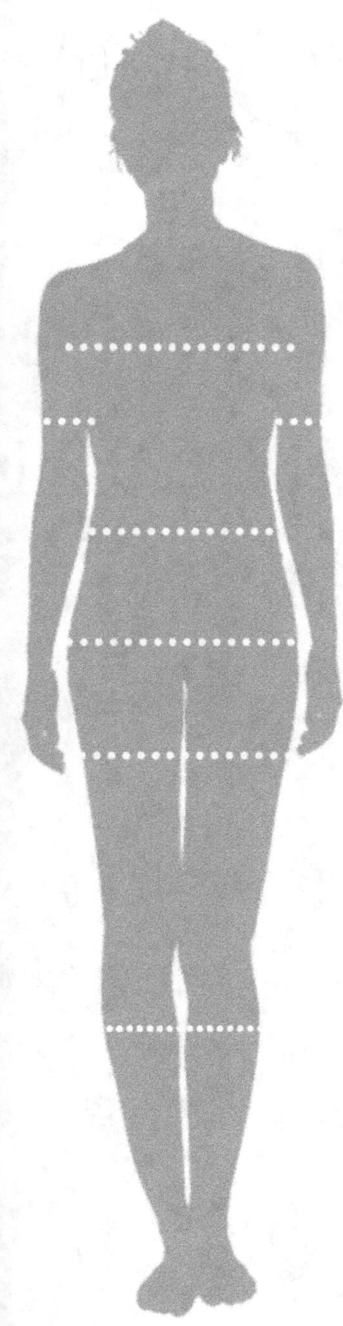

	BEFORE	AFTER
DATE		
CHEST		
LEFT ARM		
RIGHT ARM		
WAIST		
HIPS		
LEFT THIGH		
RIGHT THIGH		
LEFT CALF		
RIGHT CALF		
WEIGHT		
NOTES		

BODY MEASUREMENTS TRACKER

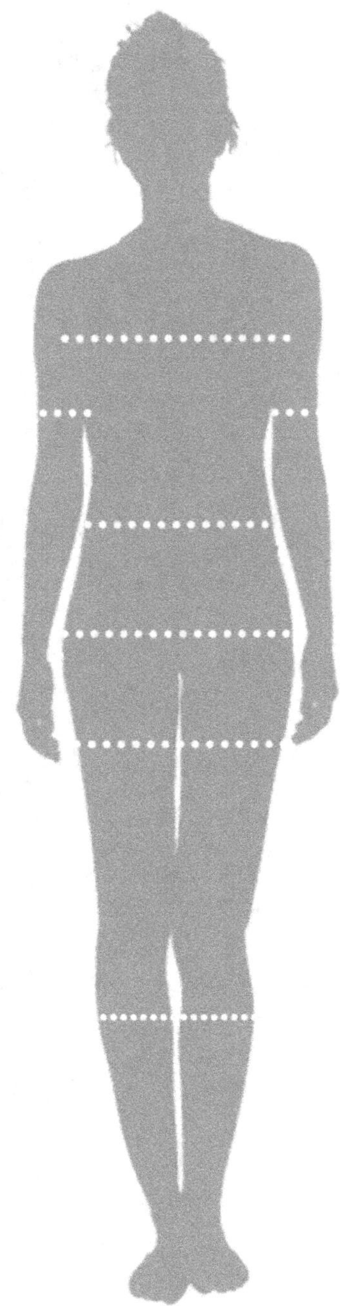

	BEFORE	AFTER
DATE		
CHEST		
LEFT ARM		
RIGHT ARM		
WAIST		
HIPS		
LEFT THIGH		
RIGHT THIGH		
LEFT CALF		
RIGHT CALF		
WEIGHT		
NOTES		

BODY MEASUREMENTS TRACKER

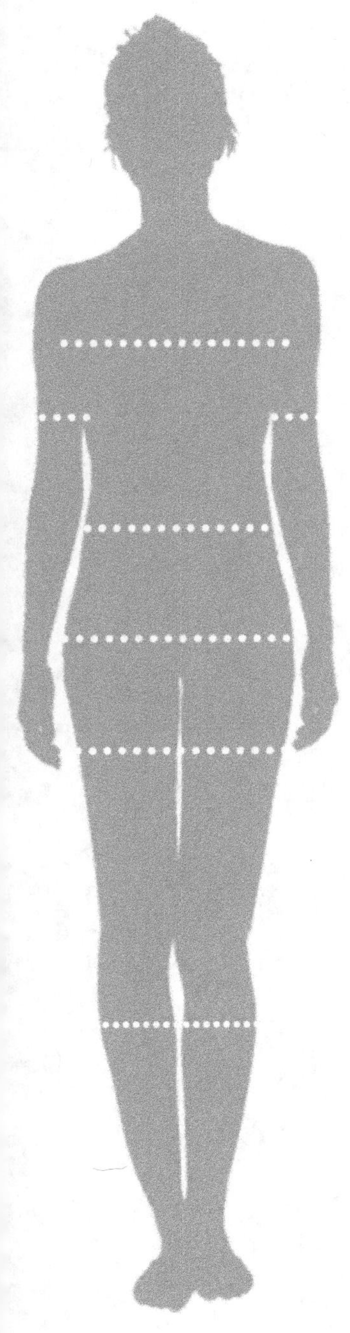

BEFORE

DATE

CHEST

LEFT ARM

RIGHT ARM

WAIST

HIPS

LEFT THIGH

RIGHT THIGH

LEFT CALF

RIGHT CALF

WEIGHT

NOTES

AFTER

DATE

CHEST

LEFT ARM

RIGHT ARM

WAIST

HIPS

LEFT THIGH

RIGHT THIGH

LEFT CALF

RIGHT CALF

WEIGHT

BODY MEASUREMENTS TRACKER

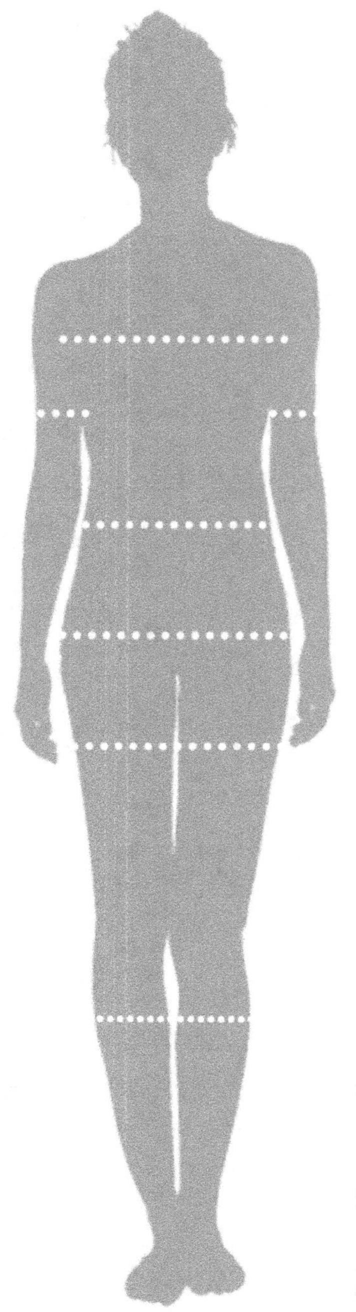

	BEFORE	AFTER
DATE		
CHEST		
LEFT ARM		
RIGHT ARM		
WAIST		
HIPS		
LEFT THIGH		
RIGHT THIGH		
LEFT CALF		
RIGHT CALF		
WEIGHT		
NOTES		

BODY MEASUREMENTS TRACKER

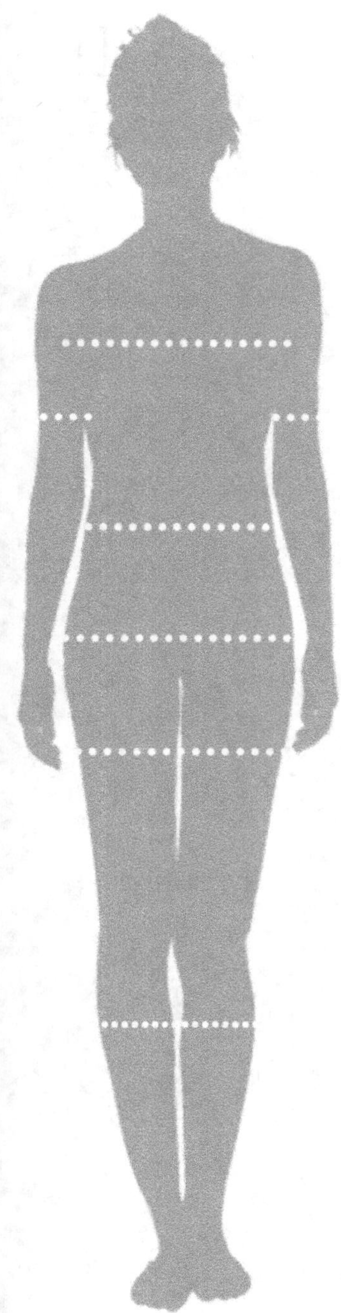

	BEFORE	AFTER
DATE		
CHEST		
LEFT ARM		
RIGHT ARM		
WAIST		
HIPS		
LEFT THIGH		
RIGHT THIGH		
LEFT CALF		
RIGHT CALF		
WEIGHT		
NOTES		

BODY MEASUREMENTS TRACKER

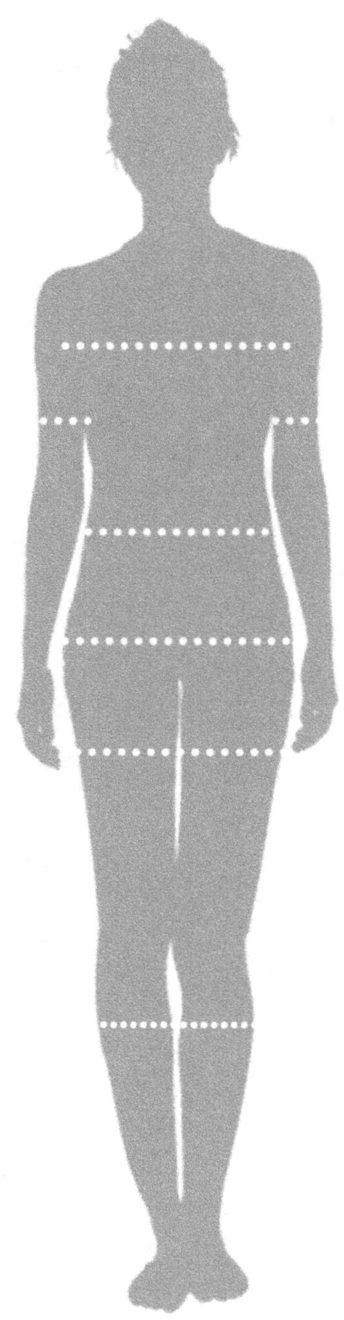

	BEFORE	AFTER
DATE		
CHEST		
LEFT ARM		
RIGHT ARM		
WAIST		
HIPS		
LEFT THIGH		
RIGHT THIGH		
LEFT CALF		
RIGHT CALF		
WEIGHT		
NOTES		

BODY MEASUREMENTS TRACKER

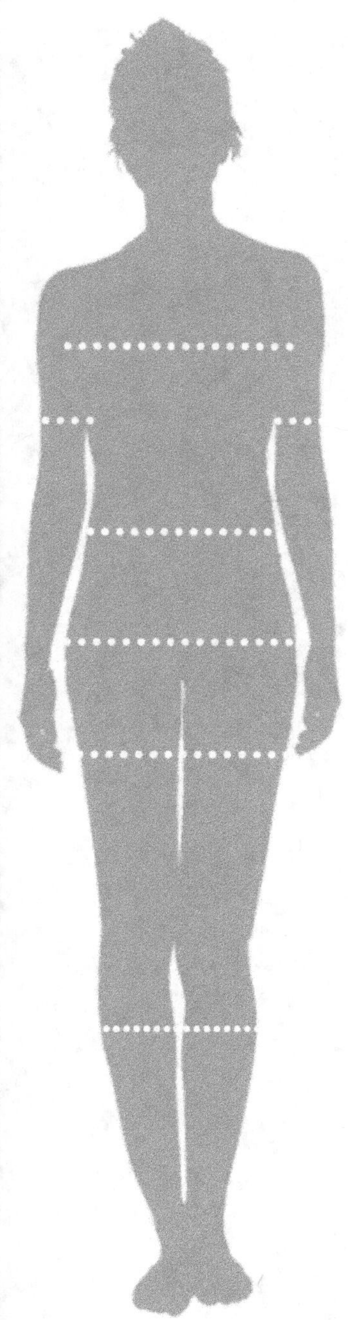

	BEFORE	AFTER
DATE		
CHEST		
LEFT ARM		
RIGHT ARM		
WAIST		
HIPS		
LEFT THIGH		
RIGHT THIGH		
LEFT CALF		
RIGHT CALF		
WEIGHT		
NOTES		

BODY MEASUREMENTS TRACKER

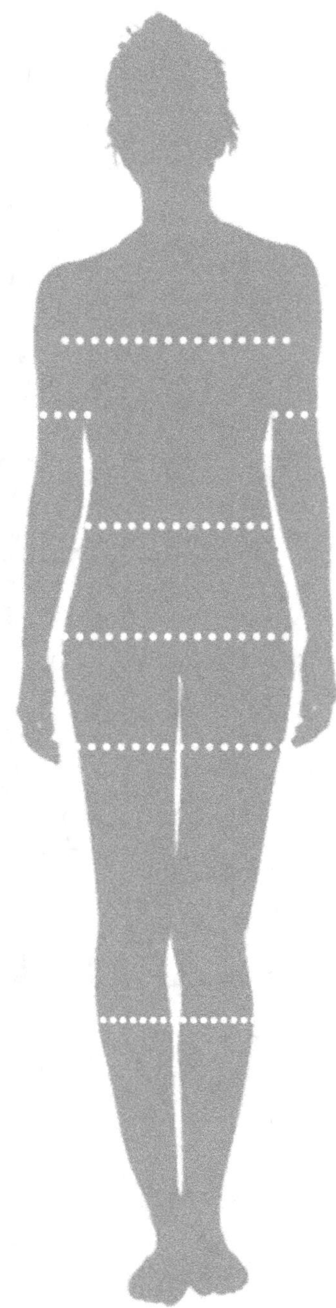

	BEFORE	AFTER
DATE		
CHEST		
LEFT ARM		
RIGHT ARM		
WAIST		
HIPS		
LEFT THIGH		
RIGHT THIGH		
LEFT CALF		
RIGHT CALF		
WEIGHT		
NOTES		

BODY MEASUREMENTS TRACKER

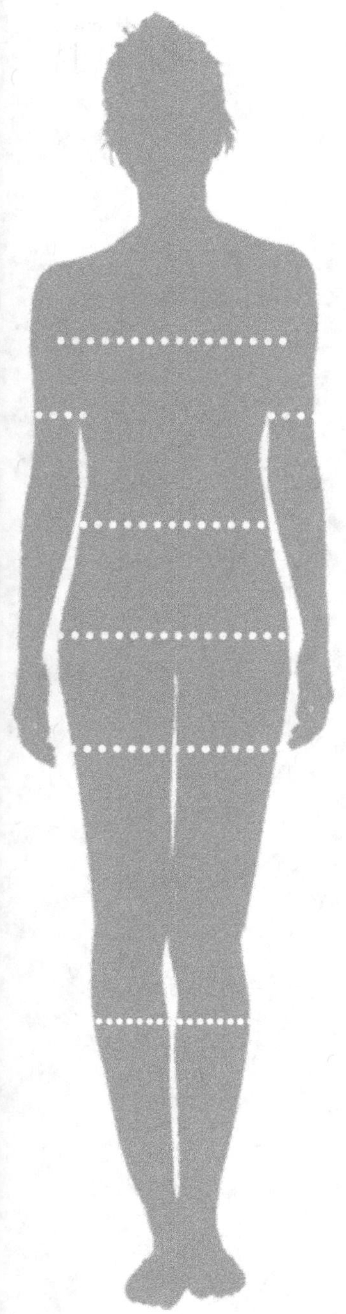

	BEFORE	AFTER
DATE		
CHEST		
LEFT ARM		
RIGHT ARM		
WAIST		
HIPS		
LEFT THIGH		
RIGHT THIGH		
LEFT CALF		
RIGHT CALF		
WEIGHT		
NOTES		

BODY MEASUREMENTS TRACKER

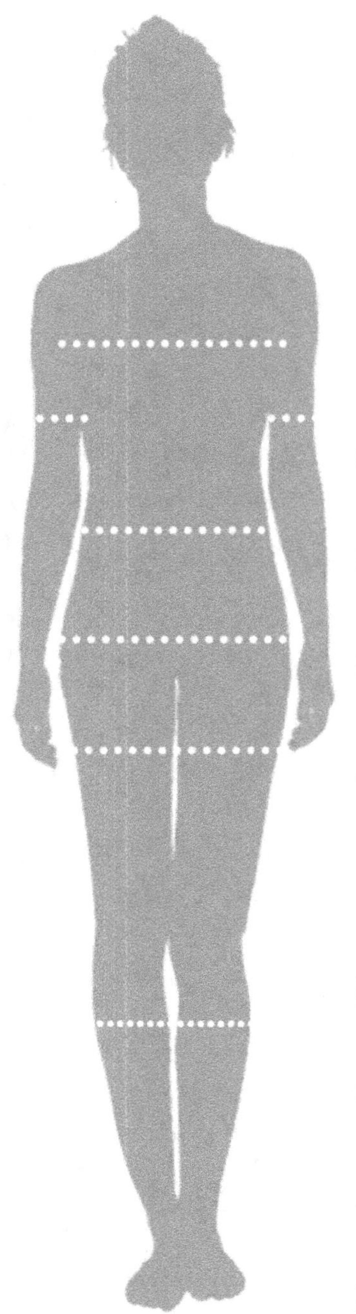

	BEFORE	AFTER
DATE		
CHEST		
LEFT ARM		
RIGHT ARM		
WAIST		
HIPS		
LEFT THIGH		
RIGHT THIGH		
LEFT CALF		
RIGHT CALF		
WEIGHT		
NOTES		

BODY MEASUREMENTS TRACKER

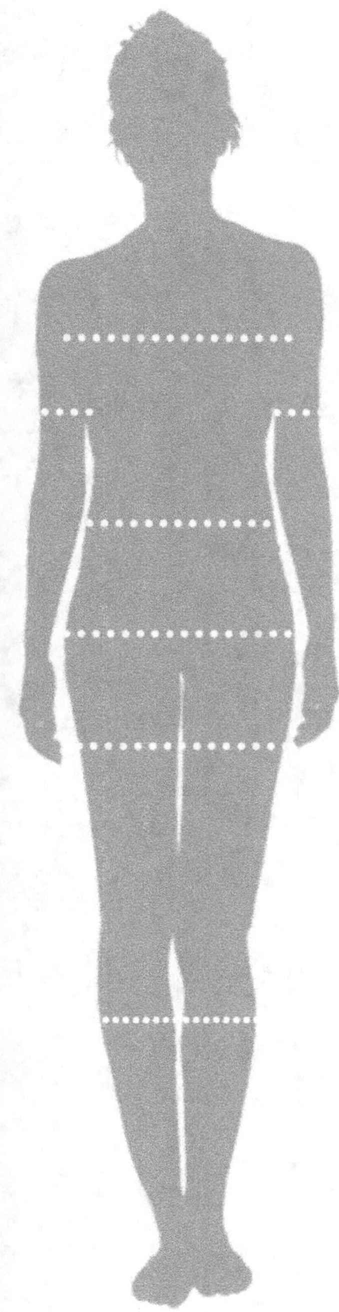

	BEFORE	AFTER
DATE		
CHEST		
LEFT ARM		
RIGHT ARM		
WAIST		
HIPS		
LEFT THIGH		
RIGHT THIGH		
LEFT CALF		
RIGHT CALF		
WEIGHT		
NOTES		

BODY MEASUREMENTS TRACKER

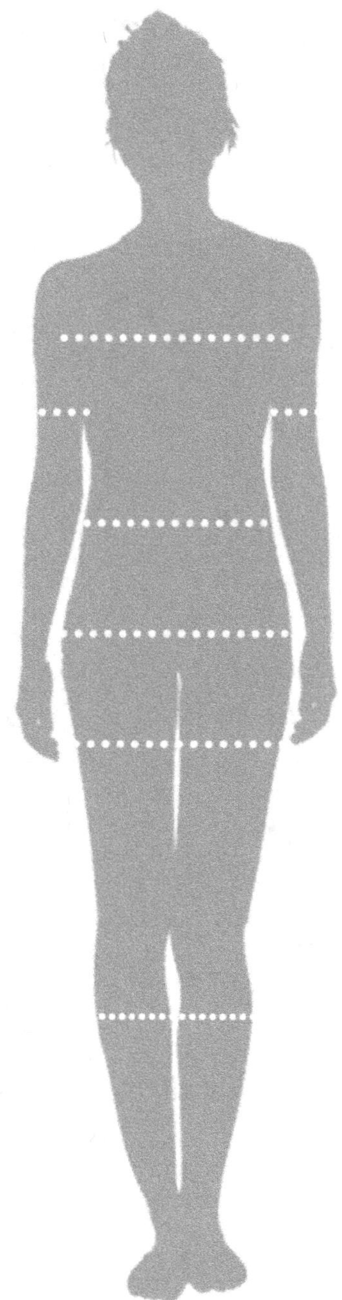

	BEFORE	AFTER
DATE		
CHEST		
LEFT ARM		
RIGHT ARM		
WAIST		
HIPS		
LEFT THIGH		
RIGHT THIGH		
LEFT CALF		
RIGHT CALF		
WEIGHT		
NOTES		

BODY MEASUREMENTS TRACKER

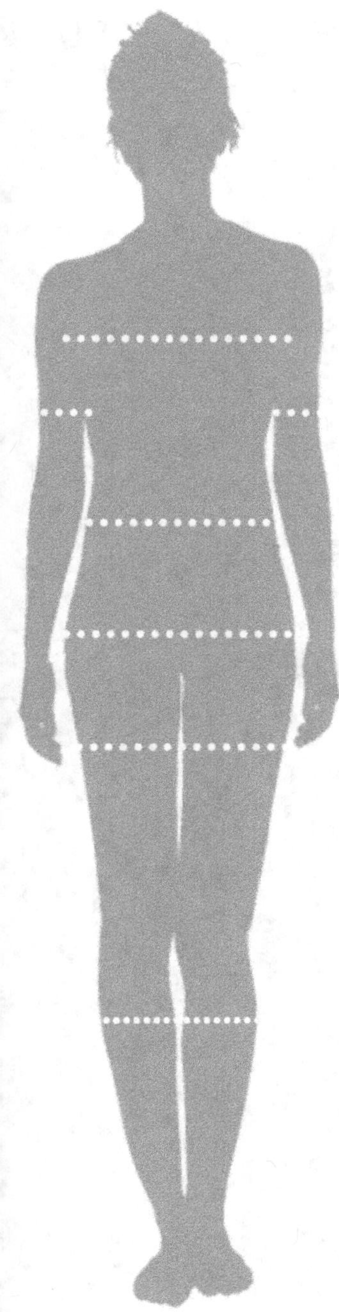

	BEFORE	AFTER
DATE		
CHEST		
LEFT ARM		
RIGHT ARM		
WAIST		
HIPS		
LEFT THIGH		
RIGHT THIGH		
LEFT CALF		
RIGHT CALF		
WEIGHT		
NOTES		

BODY MEASUREMENTS TRACKER

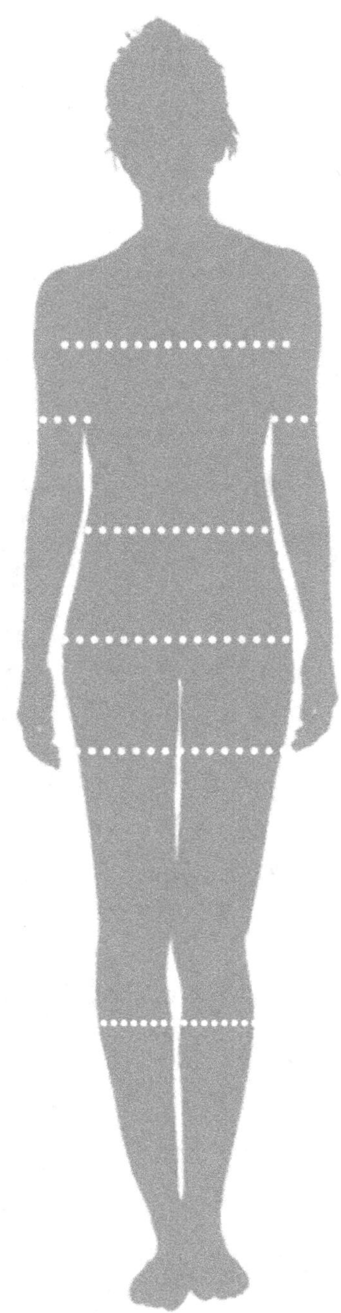

BEFORE

DATE

CHEST

LEFT ARM

RIGHT ARM

WAIST

HIPS

LEFT THIGH

RIGHT THIGH

LEFT CALF

RIGHT CALF

WEIGHT

NOTES

AFTER

DATE

CHEST

LEFT ARM

RIGHT ARM

WAIST

HIPS

LEFT THIGH

RIGHT THIGH

LEFT CALF

RIGHT CALF

WEIGHT

BODY MEASUREMENTS TRACKER

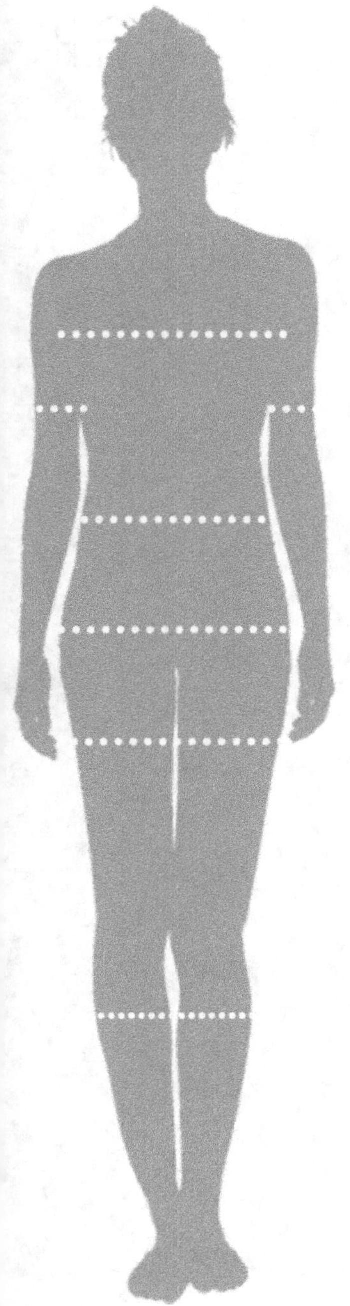

BEFORE

DATE

CHEST

LEFT ARM

RIGHT ARM

WAIST

HIPS

LEFT THIGH

RIGHT THIGH

LEFT CALF

RIGHT CALF

WEIGHT

NOTES

AFTER

DATE

CHEST

LEFT ARM

RIGHT ARM

WAIST

HIPS

LEFT THIGH

RIGHT THIGH

LEFT CALF

RIGHT CALF

WEIGHT

BODY MEASUREMENTS TRACKER

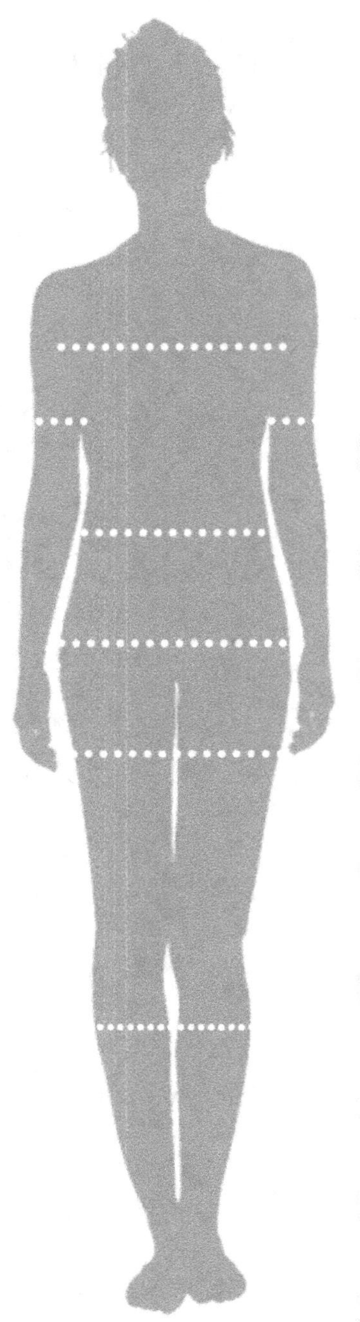

	BEFORE	AFTER
DATE		
CHEST		
LEFT ARM		
RIGHT ARM		
WAIST		
HIPS		
LEFT THIGH		
RIGHT THIGH		
LEFT CALF		
RIGHT CALF		
WEIGHT		
NOTES		

BODY MEASUREMENTS TRACKER

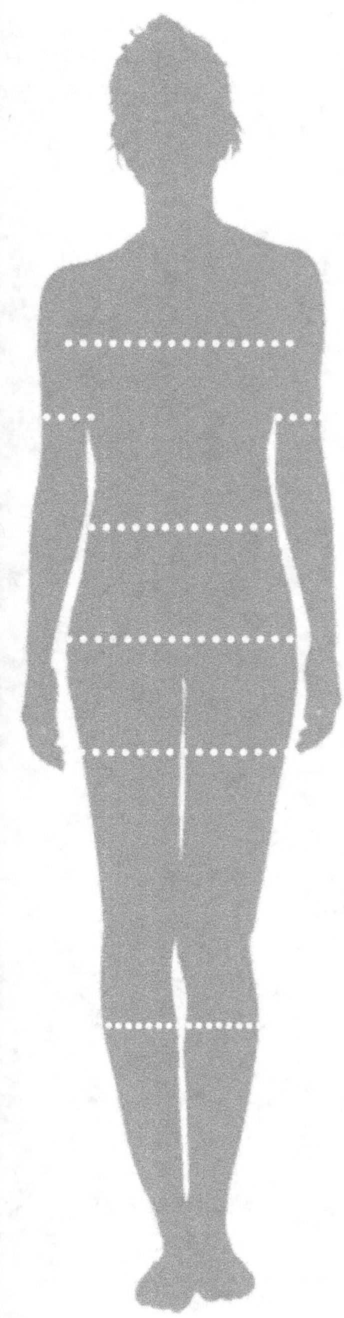

	BEFORE	AFTER
DATE		
CHEST		
LEFT ARM		
RIGHT ARM		
WAIST		
HIPS		
LEFT THIGH		
RIGHT THIGH		
LEFT CALF		
RIGHT CALF		
WEIGHT		
NOTES		

BODY MEASUREMENTS TRACKER

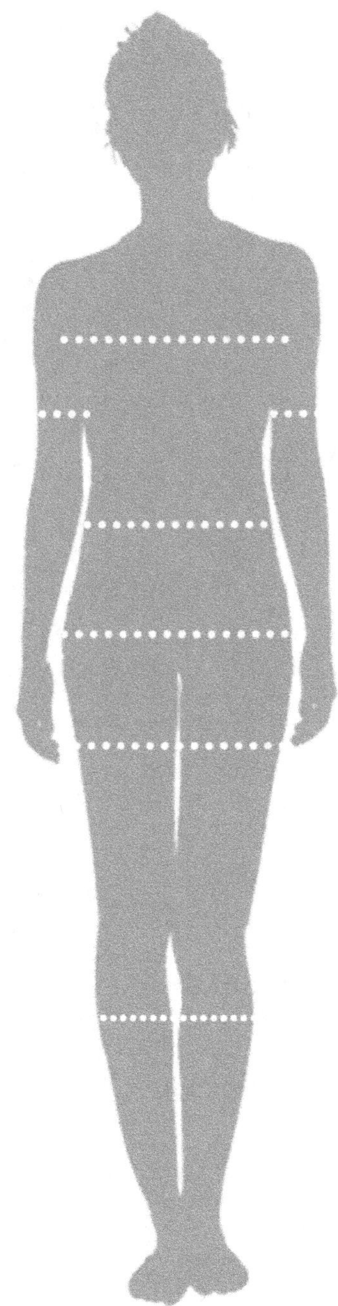

	BEFORE	AFTER
DATE		
CHEST		
LEFT ARM		
RIGHT ARM		
WAIST		
HIPS		
LEFT THIGH		
RIGHT THIGH		
LEFT CALF		
RIGHT CALF		
WEIGHT		
NOTES		

BODY MEASUREMENTS TRACKER

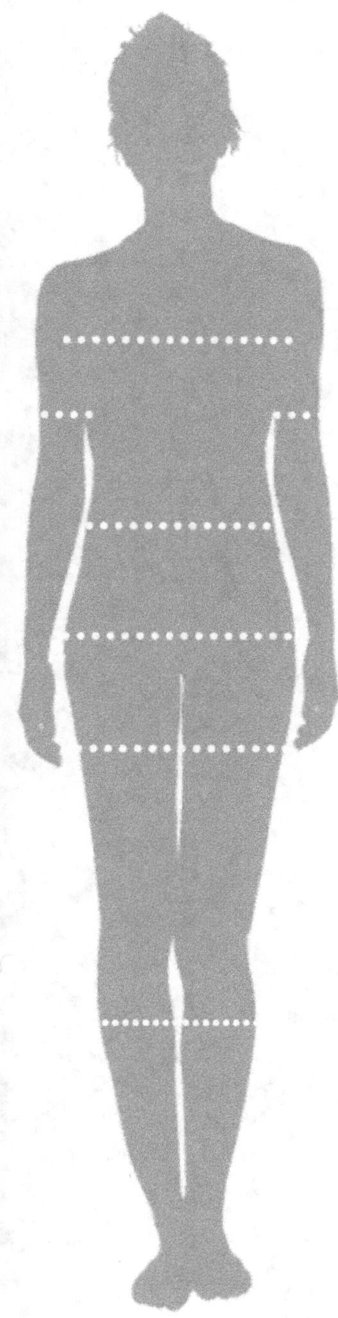

	BEFORE	AFTER
DATE		
CHEST		
LEFT ARM		
RIGHT ARM		
WAIST		
HIPS		
LEFT THIGH		
RIGHT THIGH		
LEFT CALF		
RIGHT CALF		
WEIGHT		
NOTES		

BODY MEASUREMENTS TRACKER

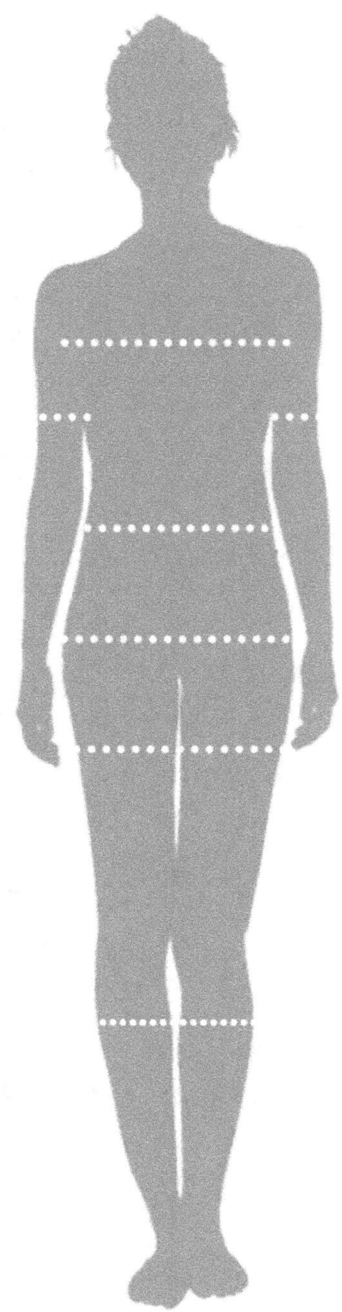

	BEFORE	AFTER
DATE		
CHEST		
LEFT ARM		
RIGHT ARM		
WAIST		
HIPS		
LEFT THIGH		
RIGHT THIGH		
LEFT CALF		
RIGHT CALF		
WEIGHT		
NOTES		

BODY MEASUREMENTS TRACKER

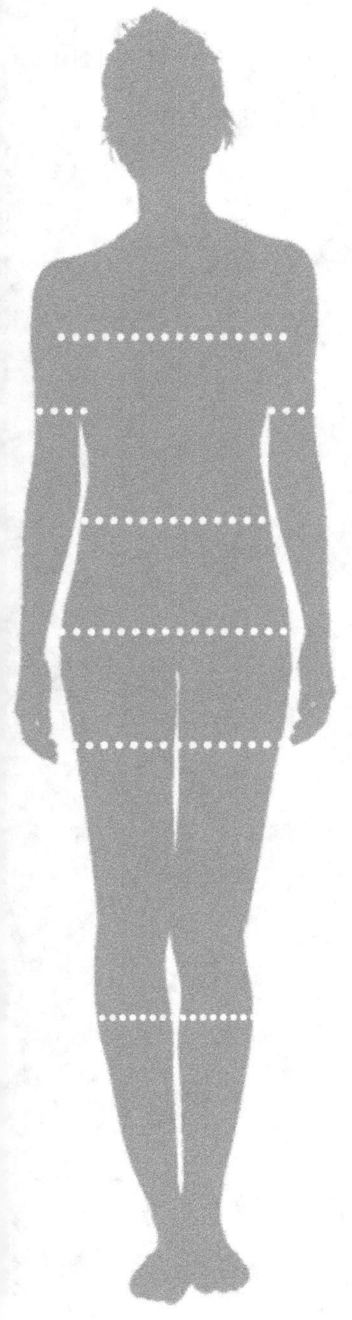

	BEFORE	AFTER
DATE		
CHEST		
LEFT ARM		
RIGHT ARM		
WAIST		
HIPS		
LEFT THIGH		
RIGHT THIGH		
LEFT CALF		
RIGHT CALF		
WEIGHT		
NOTES		

BODY MEASUREMENTS TRACKER

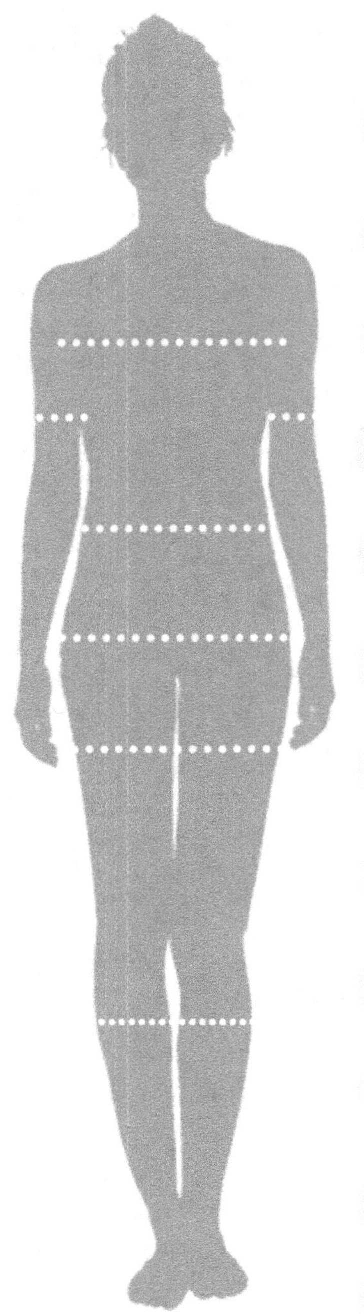

	BEFORE	AFTER
DATE		
CHEST		
LEFT ARM		
RIGHT ARM		
WAIST		
HIPS		
LEFT THIGH		
RIGHT THIGH		
LEFT CALF		
RIGHT CALF		
WEIGHT		
NOTES		

BODY MEASUREMENTS TRACKER

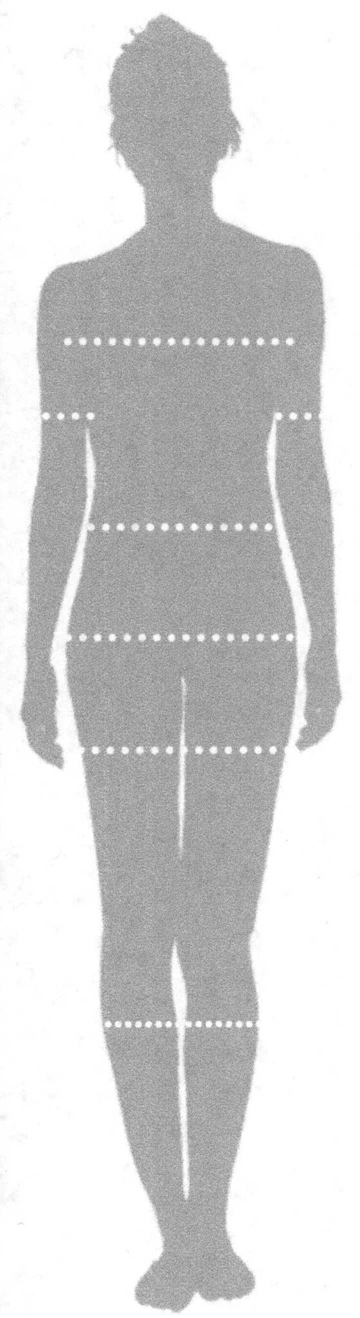

	BEFORE	AFTER
DATE		
CHEST		
LEFT ARM		
RIGHT ARM		
WAIST		
HIPS		
LEFT THIGH		
RIGHT THIGH		
LEFT CALF		
RIGHT CALF		
WEIGHT		
NOTES		

BODY MEASUREMENTS TRACKER

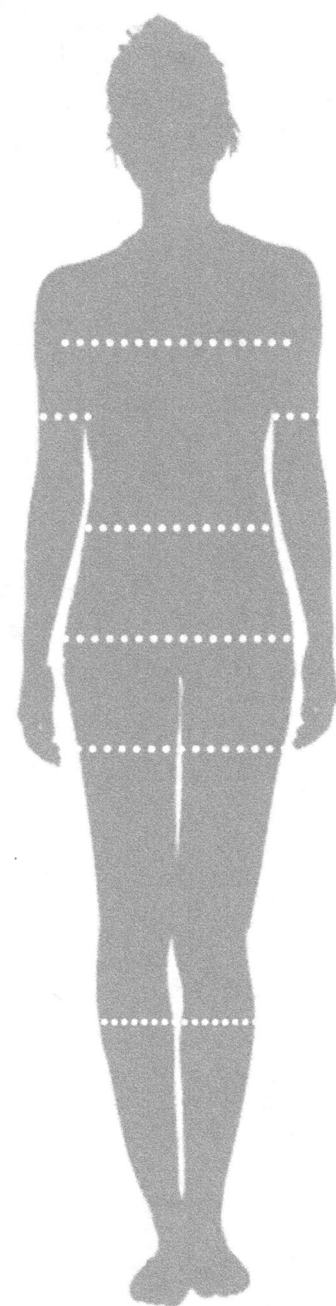

	BEFORE	AFTER
DATE		
CHEST		
LEFT ARM		
RIGHT ARM		
WAIST		
HIPS		
LEFT THIGH		
RIGHT THIGH		
LEFT CALF		
RIGHT CALF		
WEIGHT		
NOTES		

BODY MEASUREMENTS TRACKER

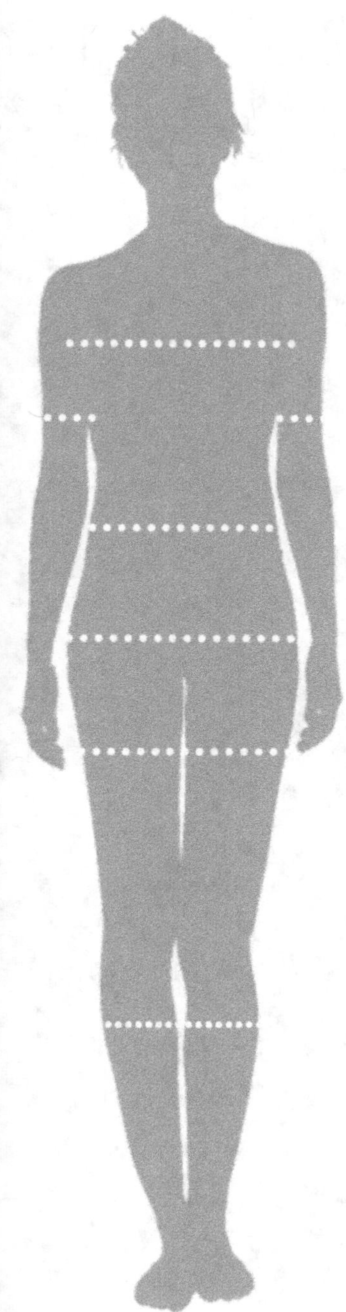

	BEFORE	AFTER
DATE		
CHEST		
LEFT ARM		
RIGHT ARM		
WAIST		
HIPS		
LEFT THIGH		
RIGHT THIGH		
LEFT CALF		
RIGHT CALF		
WEIGHT		
NOTES		

BODY MEASUREMENTS TRACKER

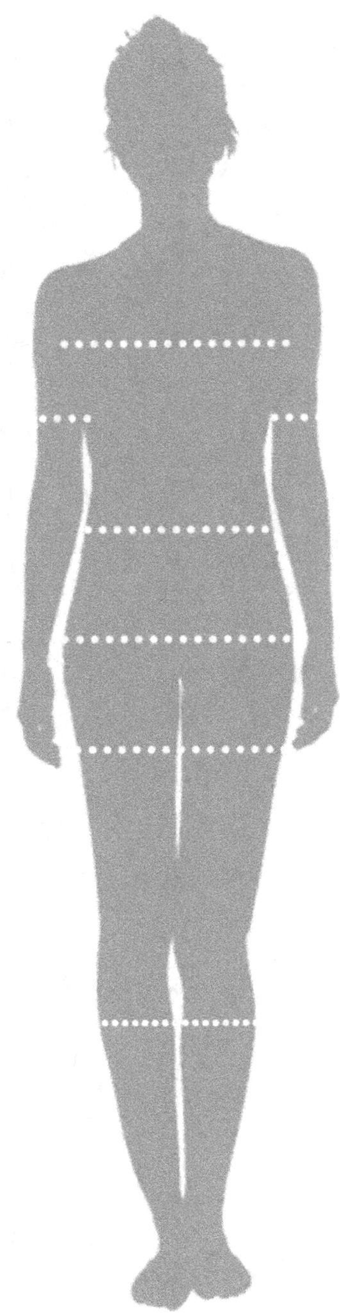

	BEFORE	AFTER
DATE		
CHEST		
LEFT ARM		
RIGHT ARM		
WAIST		
HIPS		
LEFT THIGH		
RIGHT THIGH		
LEFT CALF		
RIGHT CALF		
WEIGHT		
NOTES		

BODY MEASUREMENTS TRACKER

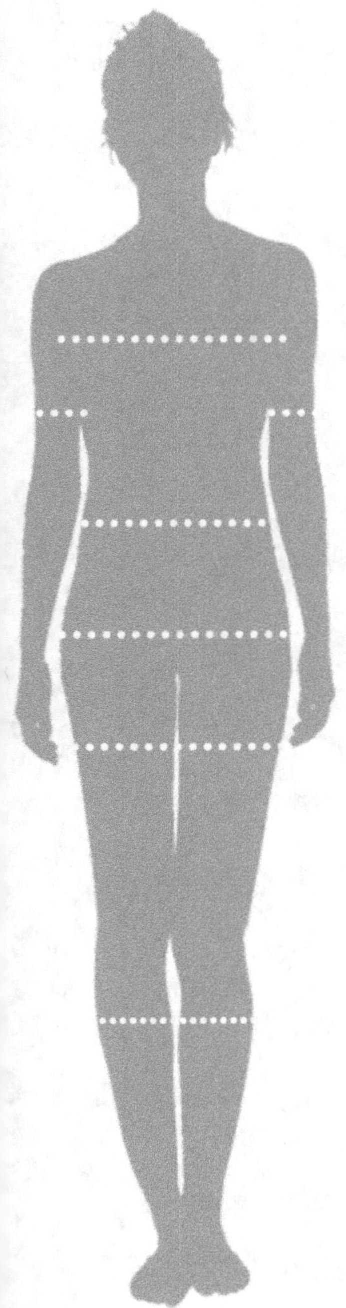

	BEFORE	AFTER
DATE		
CHEST		
LEFT ARM		
RIGHT ARM		
WAIST		
HIPS		
LEFT THIGH		
RIGHT THIGH		
LEFT CALF		
RIGHT CALF		
WEIGHT		
NOTES		

BODY MEASUREMENTS TRACKER

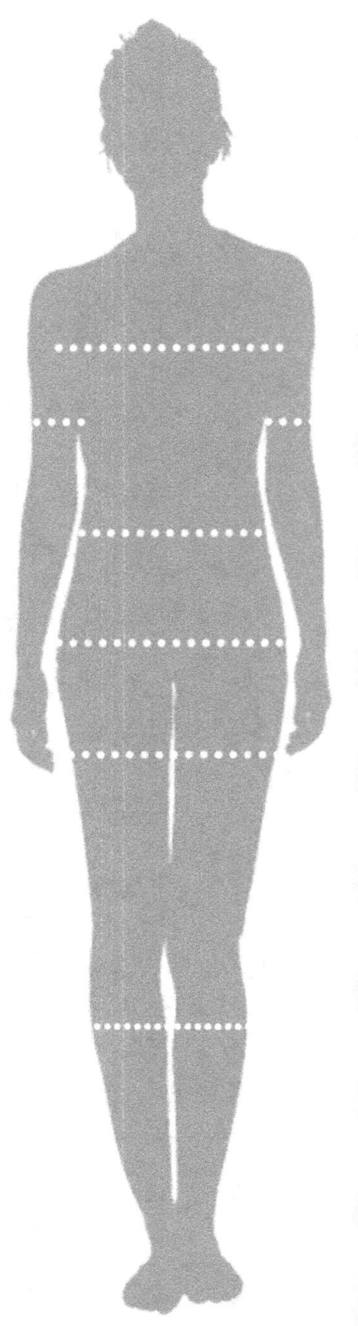

	BEFORE	AFTER
DATE		
CHEST		
LEFT ARM		
RIGHT ARM		
WAIST		
HIPS		
LEFT THIGH		
RIGHT THIGH		
LEFT CALF		
RIGHT CALF		
WEIGHT		
NOTES		

BODY MEASUREMENTS TRACKER

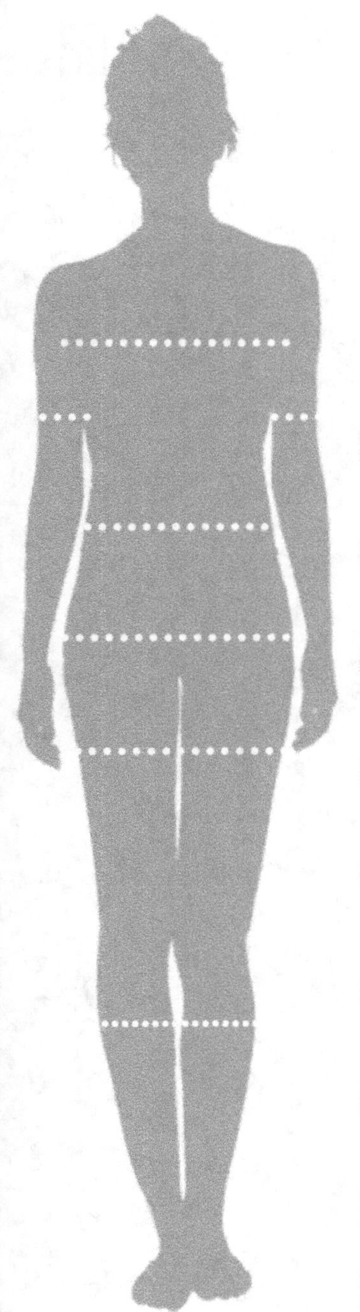

	BEFORE	AFTER
DATE		
CHEST		
LEFT ARM		
RIGHT ARM		
WAIST		
HIPS		
LEFT THIGH		
RIGHT THIGH		
LEFT CALF		
RIGHT CALF		
WEIGHT		
NOTES		

BODY MEASUREMENTS TRACKER

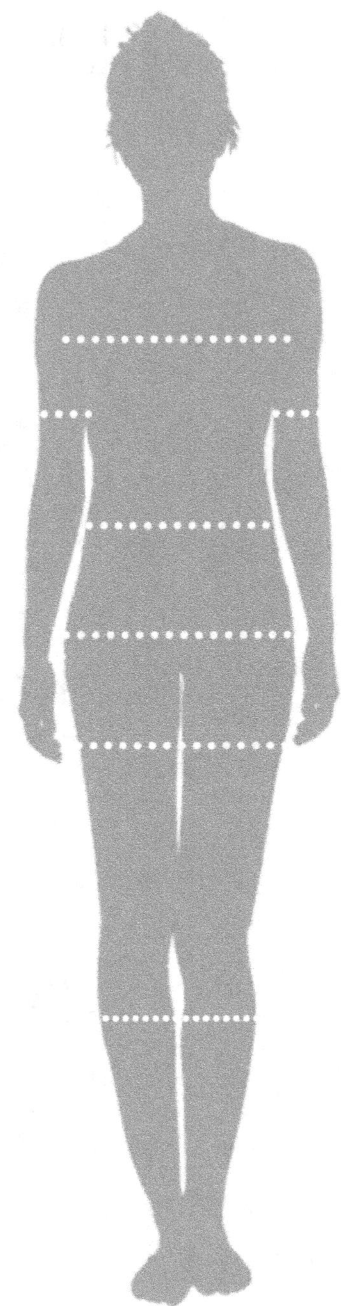

	BEFORE	AFTER
DATE		
CHEST		
LEFT ARM		
RIGHT ARM		
WAIST		
HIPS		
LEFT THIGH		
RIGHT THIGH		
LEFT CALF		
RIGHT CALF		
WEIGHT		
NOTES		

BODY MEASUREMENTS TRACKER

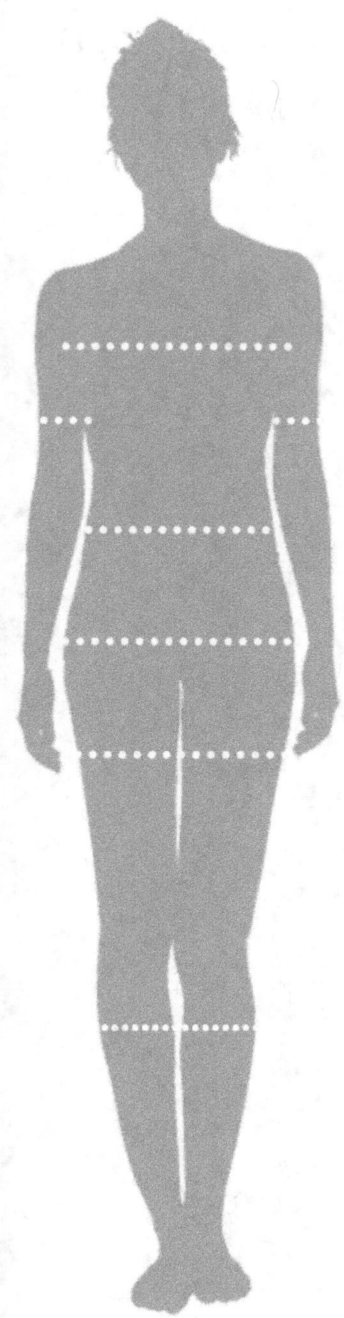

	BEFORE	AFTER
DATE		
CHEST		
LEFT ARM		
RIGHT ARM		
WAIST		
HIPS		
LEFT THIGH		
RIGHT THIGH		
LEFT CALF		
RIGHT CALF		
WEIGHT		
NOTES		

BODY MEASUREMENTS TRACKER

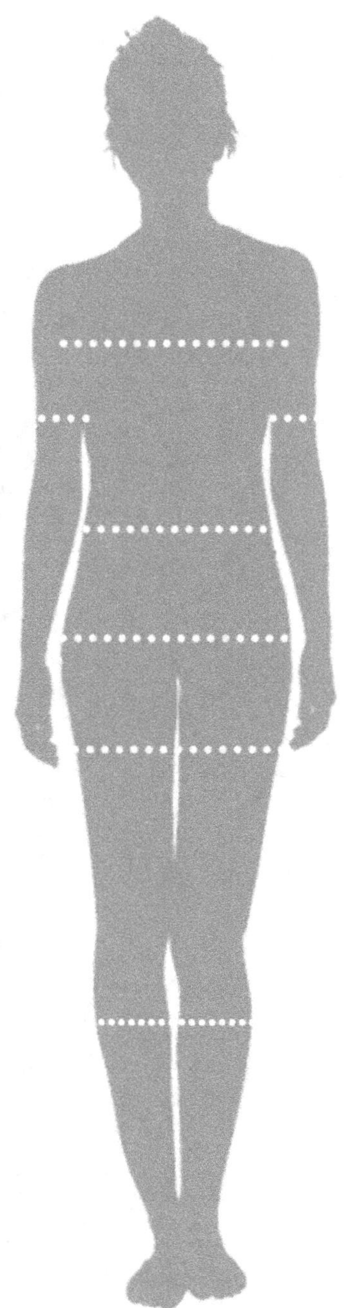

BEFORE

DATE

CHEST

LEFT ARM

RIGHT ARM

WAIST

HIPS

LEFT THIGH

RIGHT THIGH

LEFT CALF

RIGHT CALF

WEIGHT

NOTES

AFTER

DATE

CHEST

LEFT ARM

RIGHT ARM

WAIST

HIPS

LEFT THIGH

RIGHT THIGH

LEFT CALF

RIGHT CALF

WEIGHT

BODY MEASUREMENTS TRACKER

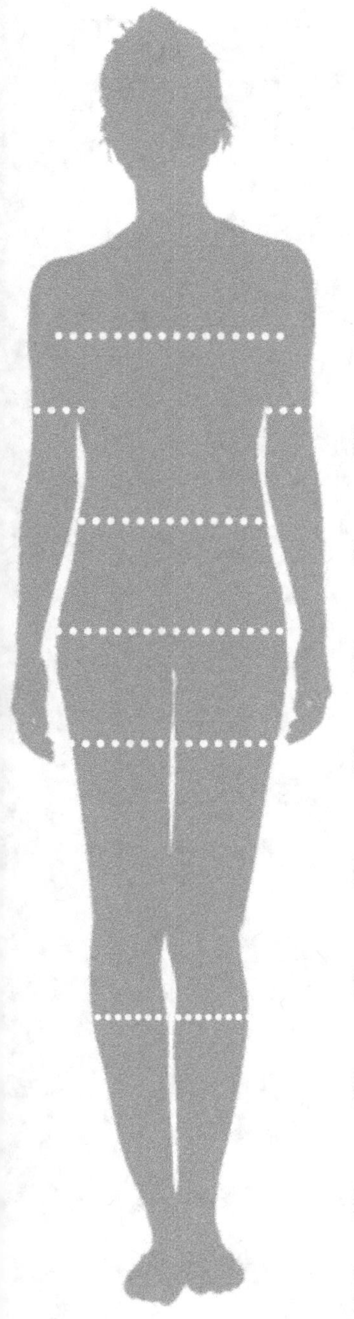

	BEFORE	AFTER
DATE		
CHEST		
LEFT ARM		
RIGHT ARM		
WAIST		
HIPS		
LEFT THIGH		
RIGHT THIGH		
LEFT CALF		
RIGHT CALF		
WEIGHT		
NOTES		

BODY MEASUREMENTS TRACKER

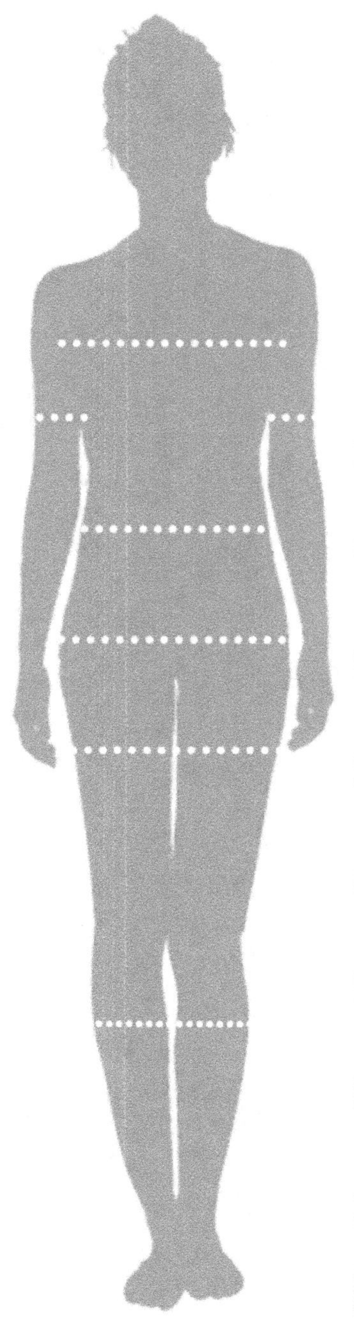

	BEFORE	AFTER
DATE		
CHEST		
LEFT ARM		
RIGHT ARM		
WAIST		
HIPS		
LEFT THIGH		
RIGHT THIGH		
LEFT CALF		
RIGHT CALF		
WEIGHT		
NOTES		

BODY MEASUREMENTS TRACKER

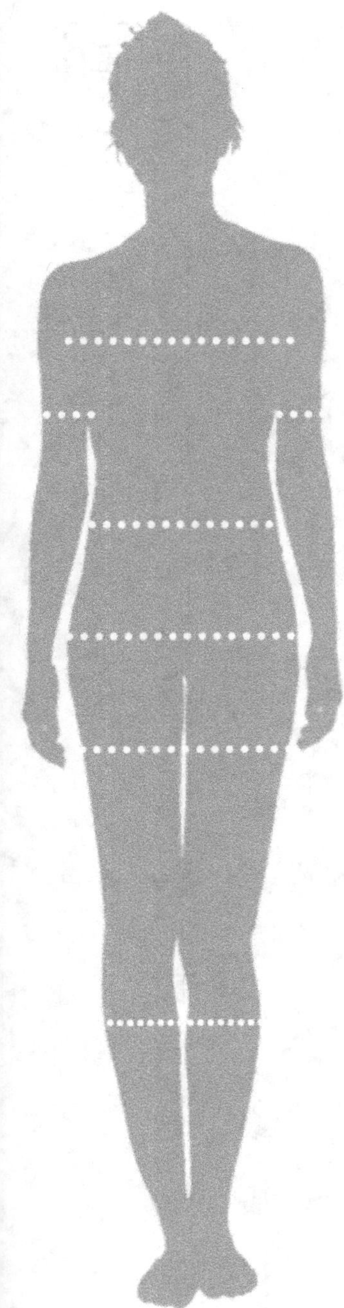

	BEFORE	AFTER
DATE		
CHEST		
LEFT ARM		
RIGHT ARM		
WAIST		
HIPS		
LEFT THIGH		
RIGHT THIGH		
LEFT CALF		
RIGHT CALF		
WEIGHT		
NOTES		

BODY MEASUREMENTS TRACKER

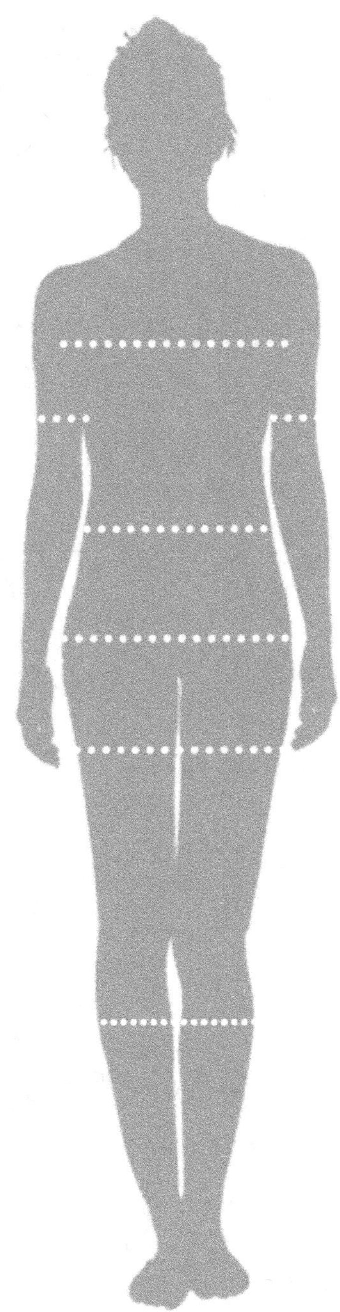

	BEFORE	AFTER
DATE		
CHEST		
LEFT ARM		
RIGHT ARM		
WAIST		
HIPS		
LEFT THIGH		
RIGHT THIGH		
LEFT CALF		
RIGHT CALF		
WEIGHT		
NOTES		

BODY MEASUREMENTS TRACKER

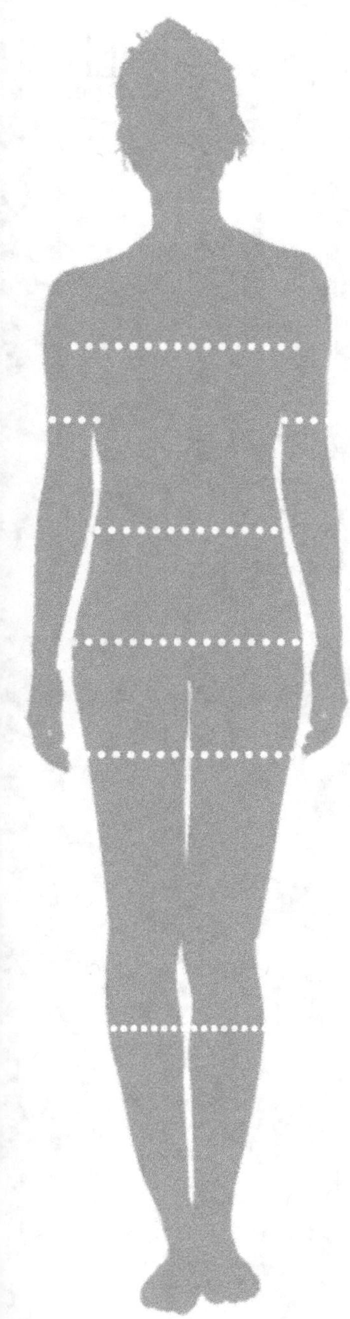

	BEFORE	AFTER
DATE		
CHEST		
LEFT ARM		
RIGHT ARM		
WAIST		
HIPS		
LEFT THIGH		
RIGHT THIGH		
LEFT CALF		
RIGHT CALF		
WEIGHT		
NOTES		

BODY MEASUREMENTS TRACKER

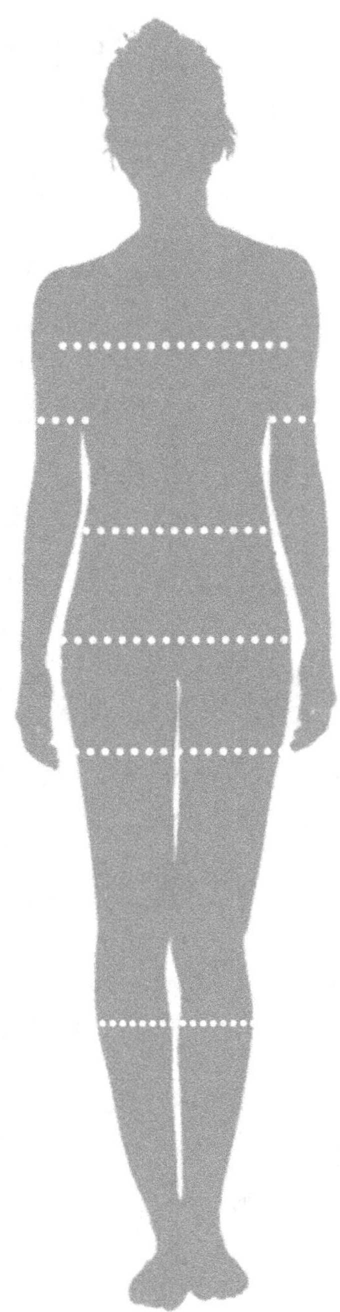

	BEFORE	AFTER
DATE		
CHEST		
LEFT ARM		
RIGHT ARM		
WAIST		
HIPS		
LEFT THIGH		
RIGHT THIGH		
LEFT CALF		
RIGHT CALF		
WEIGHT		
NOTES		

BODY MEASUREMENTS TRACKER

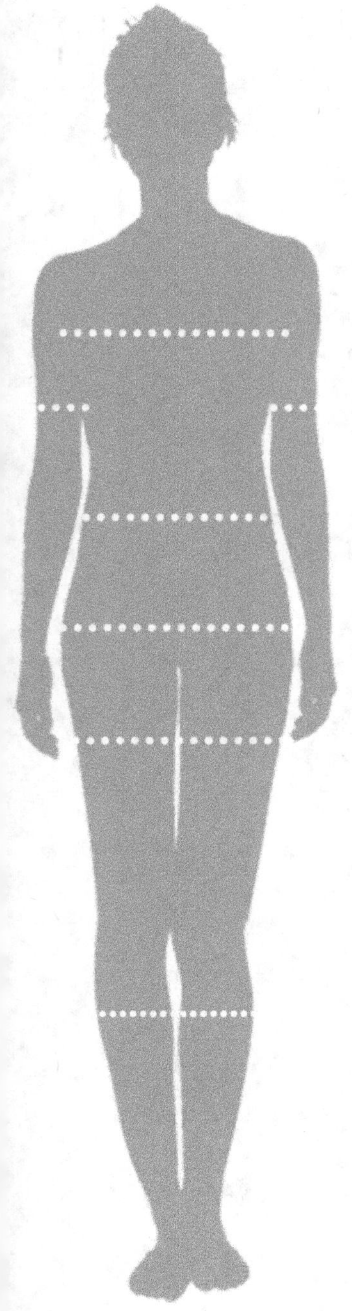

BEFORE

DATE

CHEST

LEFT ARM

RIGHT ARM

WAIST

HIPS

LEFT THIGH

RIGHT THIGH

LEFT CALF

RIGHT CALF

WEIGHT

NOTES

AFTER

DATE

CHEST

LEFT ARM

RIGHT ARM

WAIST

HIPS

LEFT THIGH

RIGHT THIGH

LEFT CALF

RIGHT CALF

WEIGHT

BODY MEASUREMENTS TRACKER

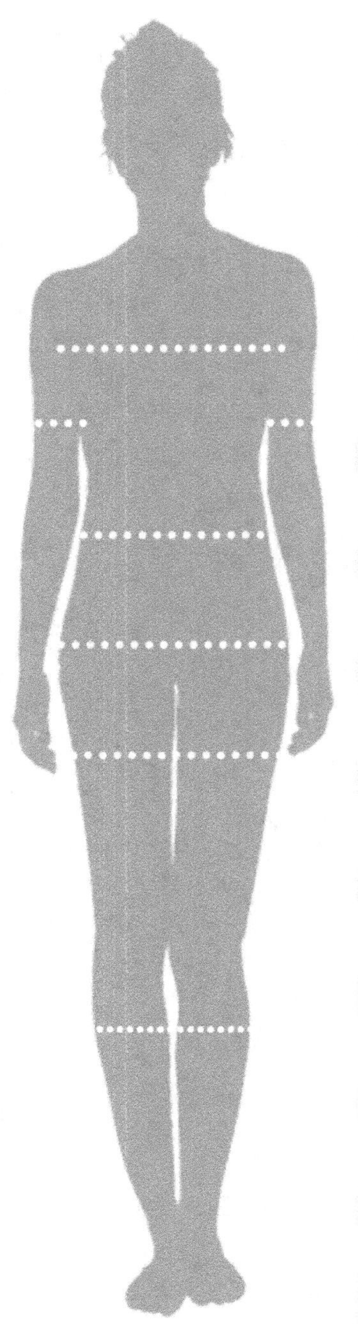

	BEFORE	AFTER
DATE		
CHEST		
LEFT ARM		
RIGHT ARM		
WAIST		
HIPS		
LEFT THIGH		
RIGHT THIGH		
LEFT CALF		
RIGHT CALF		
WEIGHT		
NOTES		

BODY MEASUREMENTS TRACKER

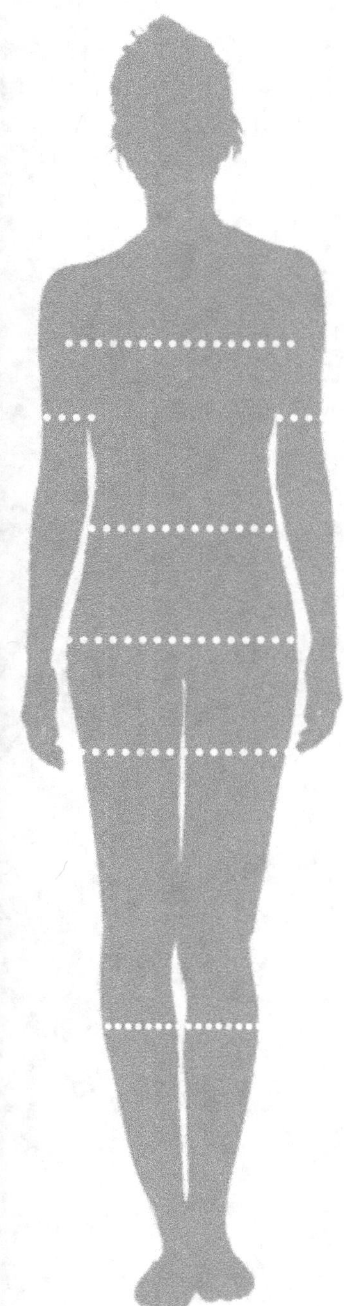

	BEFORE	AFTER
DATE		
CHEST		
LEFT ARM		
RIGHT ARM		
WAIST		
HIPS		
LEFT THIGH		
RIGHT THIGH		
LEFT CALF		
RIGHT CALF		
WEIGHT		
NOTES		

BODY MEASUREMENTS TRACKER

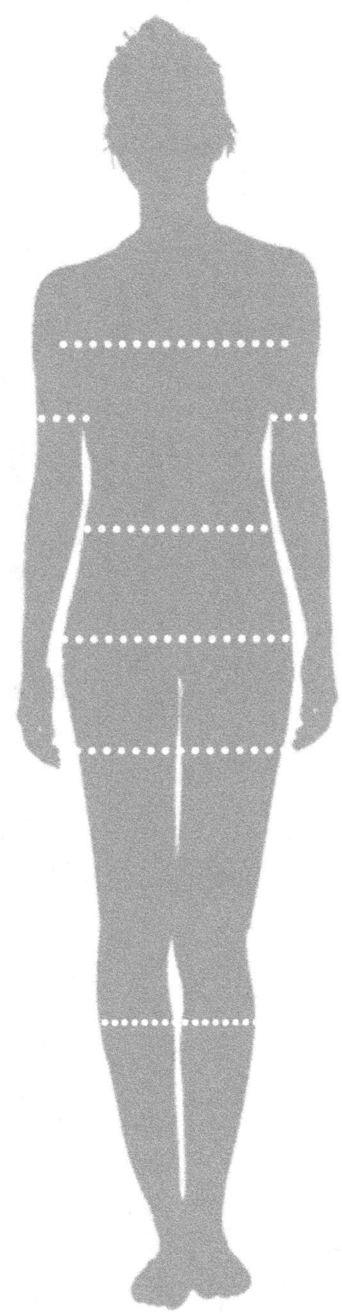

	BEFORE	AFTER
DATE		
CHEST		
LEFT ARM		
RIGHT ARM		
WAIST		
HIPS		
LEFT THIGH		
RIGHT THIGH		
LEFT CALF		
RIGHT CALF		
WEIGHT		
NOTES		

BODY MEASUREMENTS TRACKER

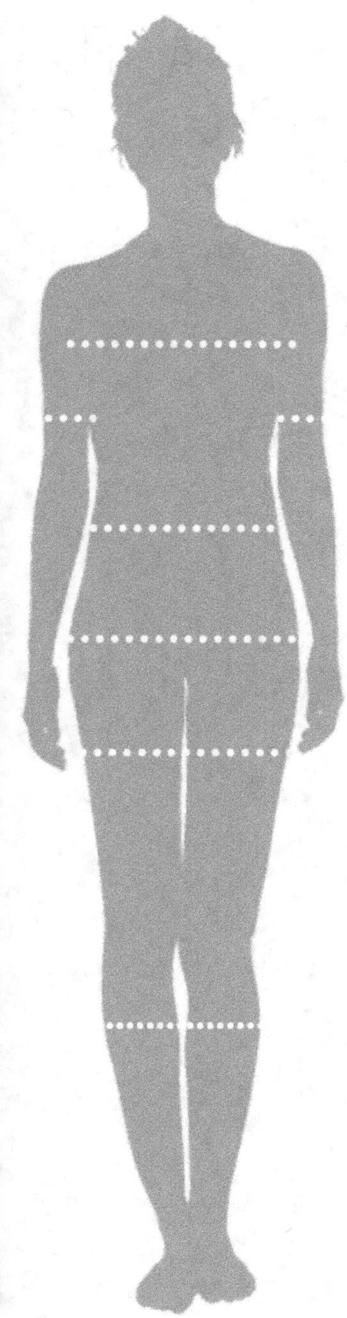

	BEFORE	AFTER
DATE		
CHEST		
LEFT ARM		
RIGHT ARM		
WAIST		
HIPS		
LEFT THIGH		
RIGHT THIGH		
LEFT CALF		
RIGHT CALF		
WEIGHT		
NOTES		

BODY MEASUREMENTS TRACKER

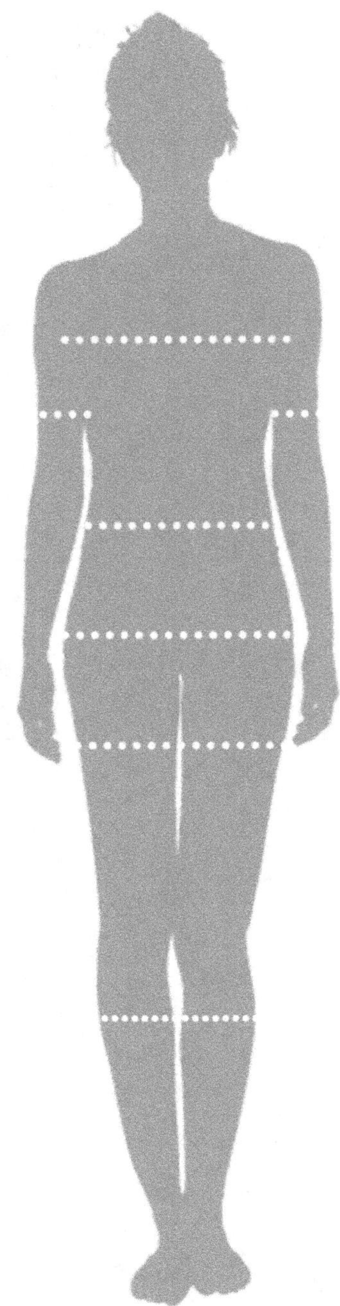

	BEFORE	AFTER
DATE		
CHEST		
LEFT ARM		
RIGHT ARM		
WAIST		
HIPS		
LEFT THIGH		
RIGHT THIGH		
LEFT CALF		
RIGHT CALF		
WEIGHT		
NOTES		

BODY MEASUREMENTS TRACKER

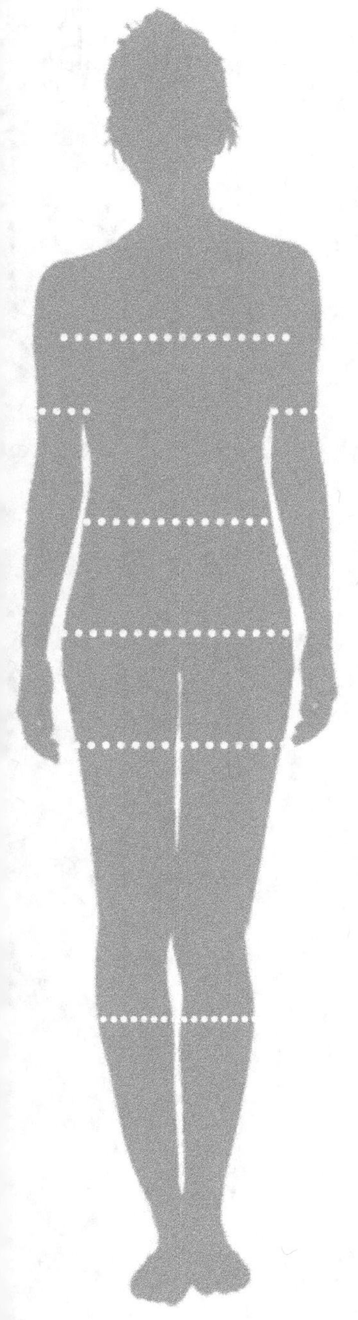

BEFORE

DATE

CHEST

LEFT ARM

RIGHT ARM

WAIST

HIPS

LEFT THIGH

RIGHT THIGH

LEFT CALF

RIGHT CALF

WEIGHT

NOTES

AFTER

DATE

CHEST

LEFT ARM

RIGHT ARM

WAIST

HIPS

LEFT THIGH

RIGHT THIGH

LEFT CALF

RIGHT CALF

WEIGHT

BODY MEASUREMENTS TRACKER

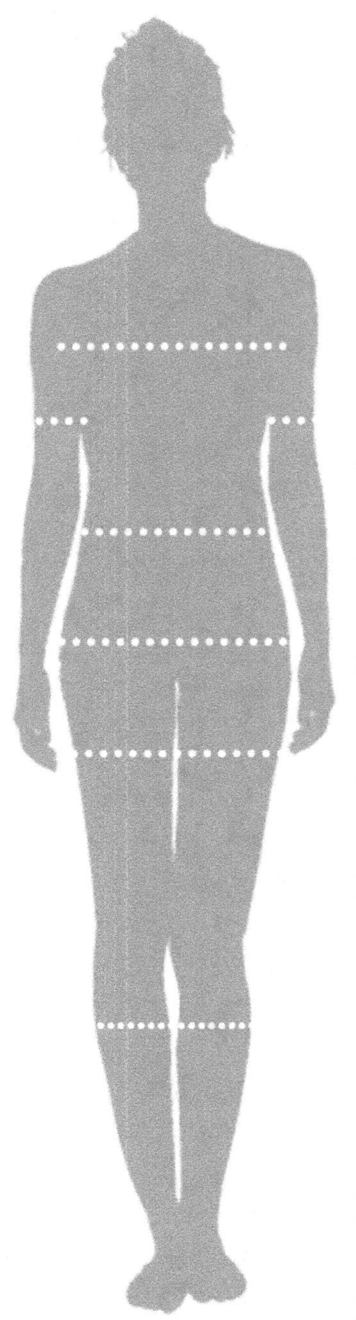

	BEFORE	AFTER
DATE		
CHEST		
LEFT ARM		
RIGHT ARM		
WAIST		
HIPS		
LEFT THIGH		
RIGHT THIGH		
LEFT CALF		
RIGHT CALF		
WEIGHT		
NOTES		

BODY MEASUREMENTS TRACKER

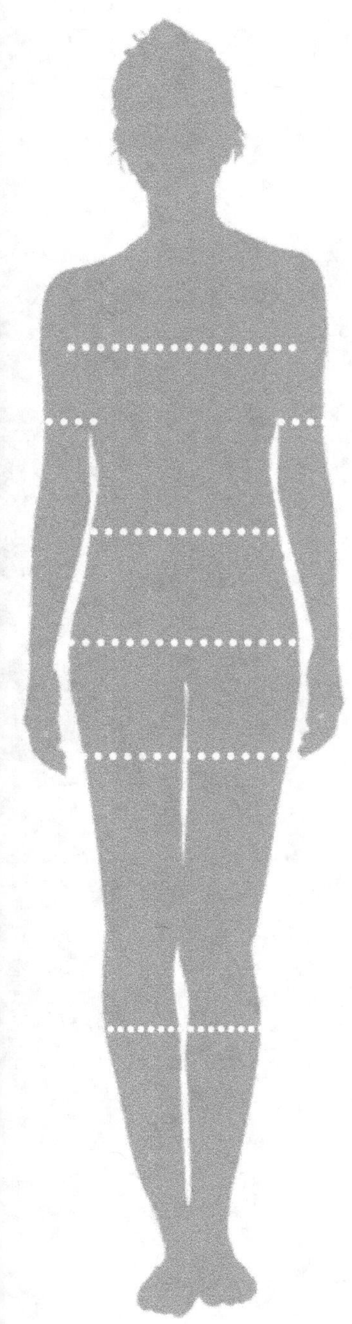

	BEFORE	AFTER
DATE		
CHEST		
LEFT ARM		
RIGHT ARM		
WAIST		
HIPS		
LEFT THIGH		
RIGHT THIGH		
LEFT CALF		
RIGHT CALF		
WEIGHT		
NOTES		

BODY MEASUREMENTS TRACKER

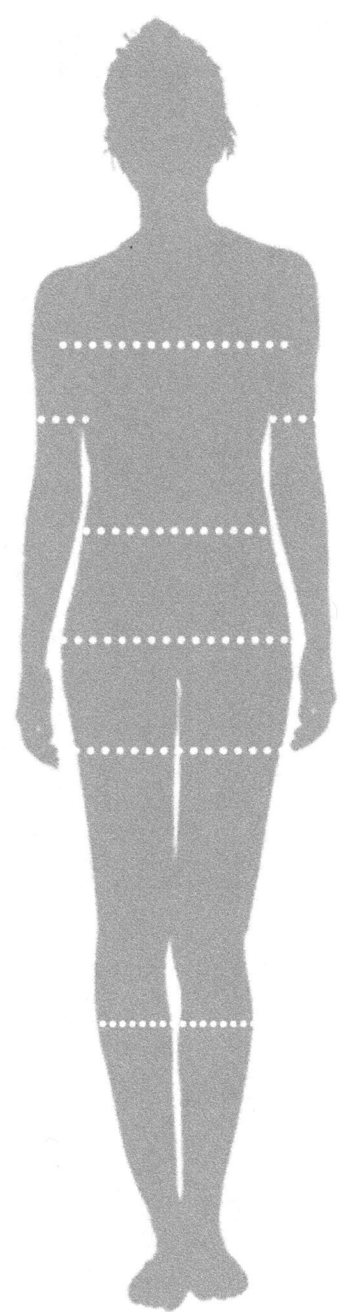

	BEFORE	AFTER
DATE		
CHEST		
LEFT ARM		
RIGHT ARM		
WAIST		
HIPS		
LEFT THIGH		
RIGHT THIGH		
LEFT CALF		
RIGHT CALF		
WEIGHT		
NOTES		

BODY MEASUREMENTS TRACKER

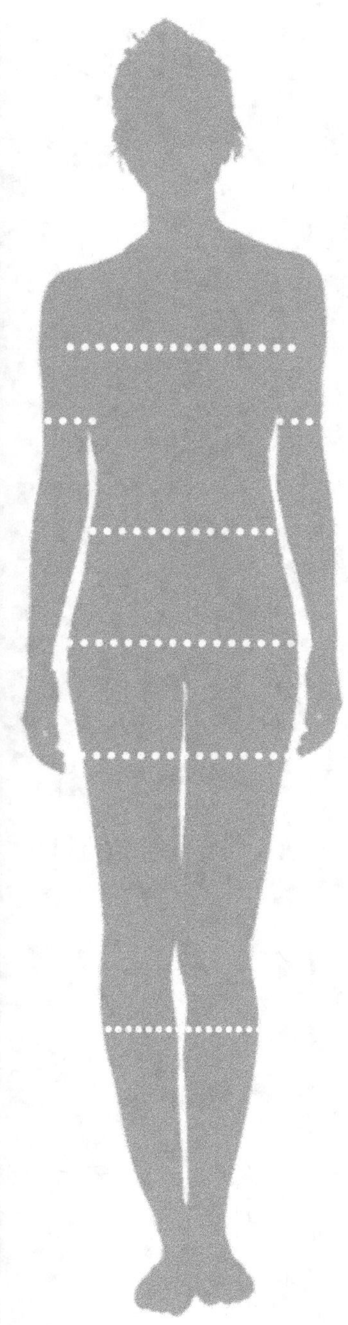

	BEFORE	AFTER
DATE		
CHEST		
LEFT ARM		
RIGHT ARM		
WAIST		
HIPS		
LEFT THIGH		
RIGHT THIGH		
LEFT CALF		
RIGHT CALF		
WEIGHT		
NOTES		

BODY MEASUREMENTS TRACKER

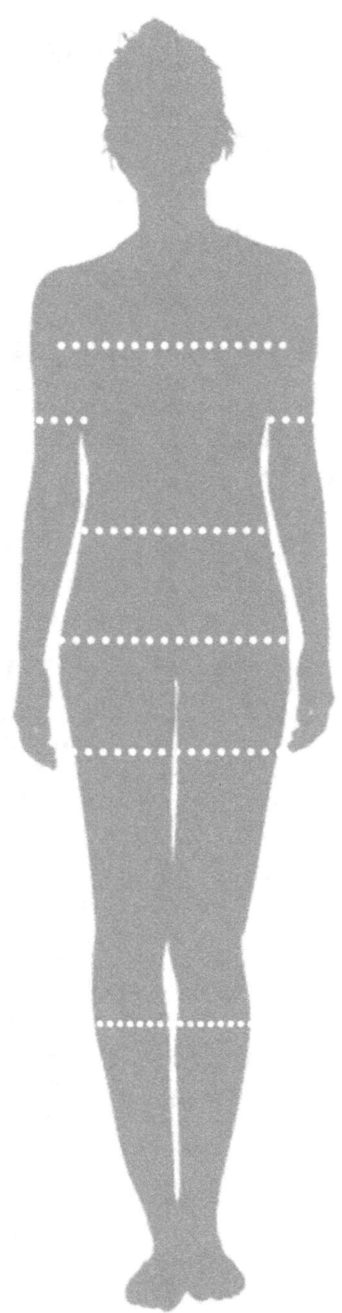

	BEFORE	AFTER
DATE		
CHEST		
LEFT ARM		
RIGHT ARM		
WAIST		
HIPS		
LEFT THIGH		
RIGHT THIGH		
LEFT CALF		
RIGHT CALF		
WEIGHT		
NOTES		

BODY MEASUREMENTS TRACKER

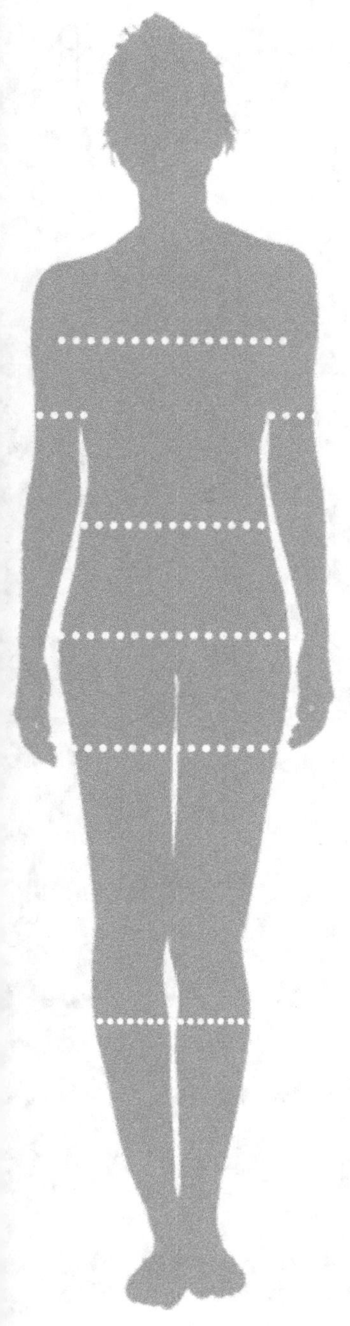

	BEFORE	AFTER
DATE		
CHEST		
LEFT ARM		
RIGHT ARM		
WAIST		
HIPS		
LEFT THIGH		
RIGHT THIGH		
LEFT CALF		
RIGHT CALF		
WEIGHT		
NOTES		

BODY MEASUREMENTS TRACKER

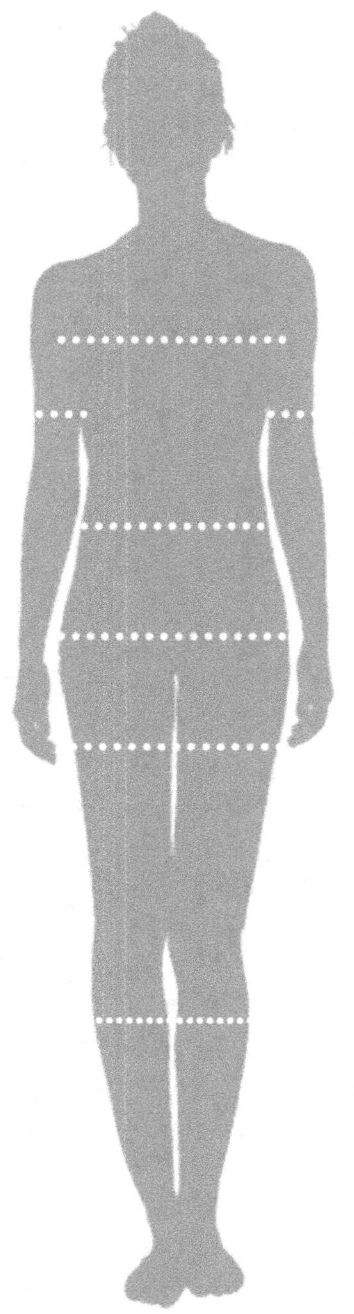

	BEFORE	AFTER
DATE		
CHEST		
LEFT ARM		
RIGHT ARM		
WAIST		
HIPS		
LEFT THIGH		
RIGHT THIGH		
LEFT CALF		
RIGHT CALF		
WEIGHT		
NOTES		

BODY MEASUREMENTS TRACKER

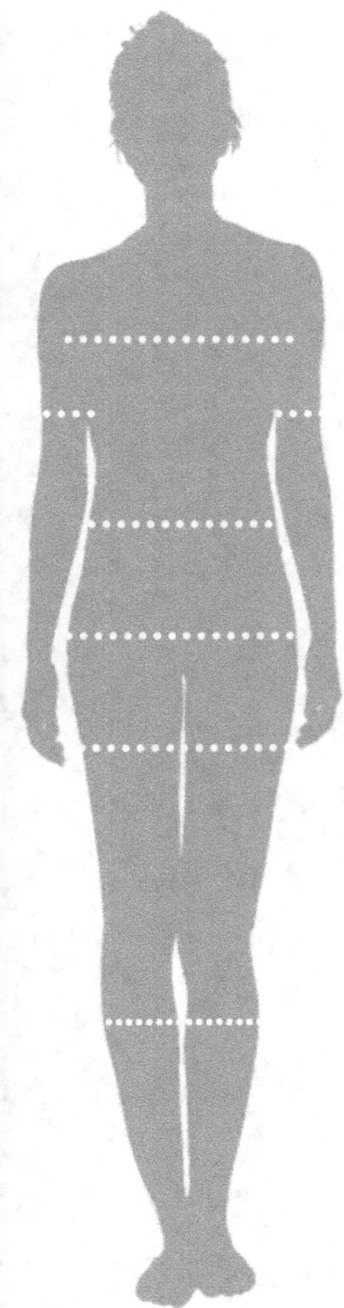

	BEFORE	AFTER
DATE		
CHEST		
LEFT ARM		
RIGHT ARM		
WAIST		
HIPS		
LEFT THIGH		
RIGHT THIGH		
LEFT CALF		
RIGHT CALF		
WEIGHT		
NOTES		

BODY MEASUREMENTS TRACKER

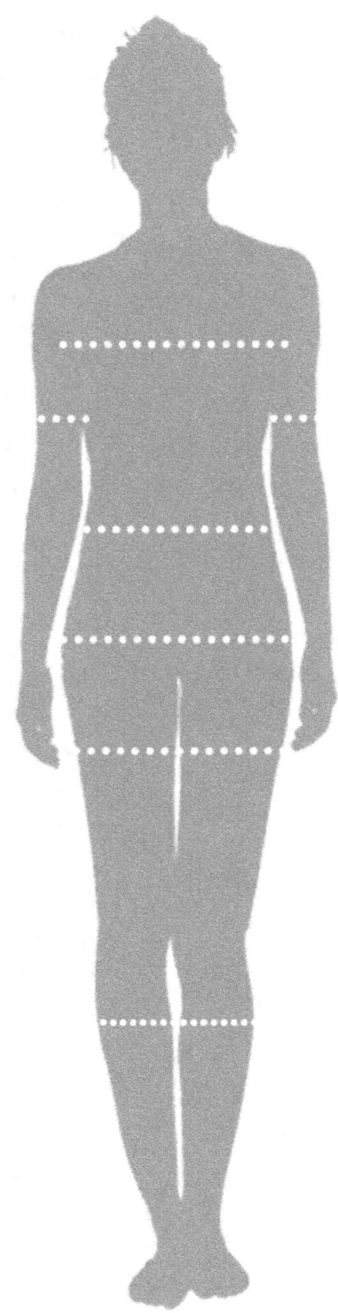

	BEFORE	AFTER
DATE		
CHEST		
LEFT ARM		
RIGHT ARM		
WAIST		
HIPS		
LEFT THIGH		
RIGHT THIGH		
LEFT CALF		
RIGHT CALF		
WEIGHT		
NOTES		

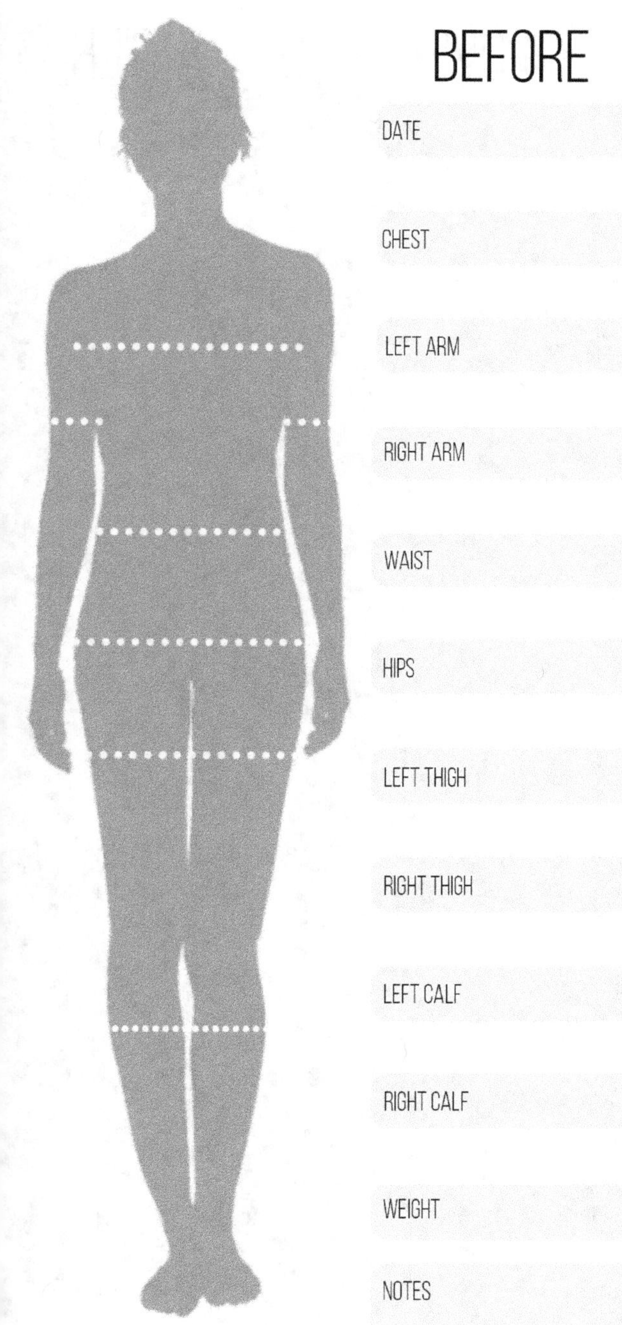

BODY MEASUREMENTS TRACKER

	BEFORE	AFTER
DATE		
CHEST		
LEFT ARM		
RIGHT ARM		
WAIST		
HIPS		
LEFT THIGH		
RIGHT THIGH		
LEFT CALF		
RIGHT CALF		
WEIGHT		
NOTES		

BODY MEASUREMENTS TRACKER

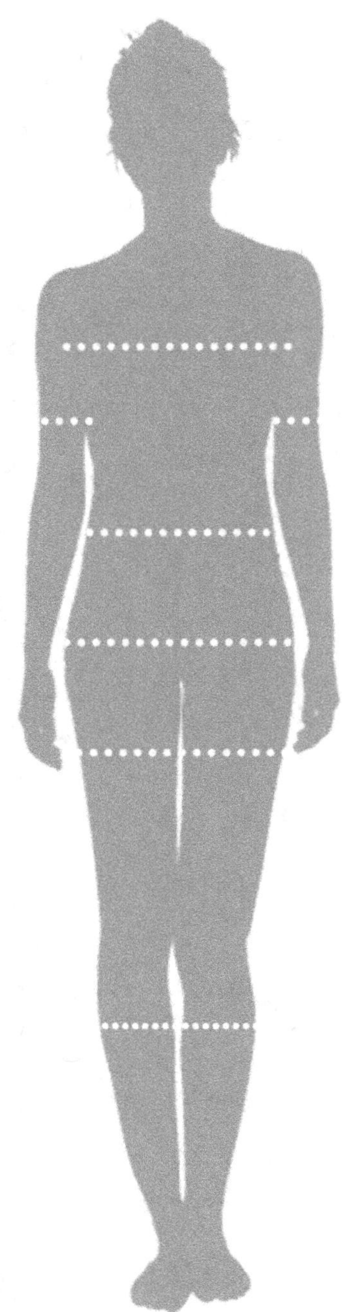

	BEFORE	AFTER
DATE		
CHEST		
LEFT ARM		
RIGHT ARM		
WAIST		
HIPS		
LEFT THIGH		
RIGHT THIGH		
LEFT CALF		
RIGHT CALF		
WEIGHT		
NOTES		

BODY MEASUREMENTS TRACKER

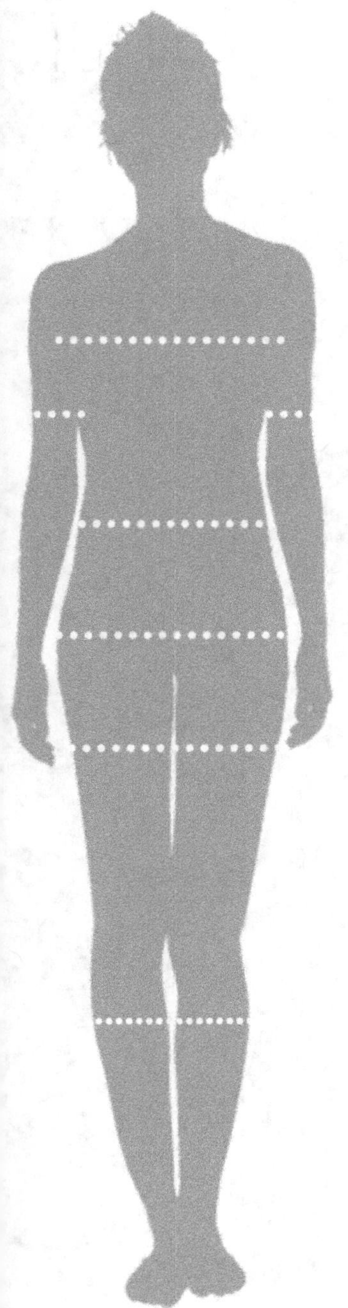

	BEFORE	AFTER
DATE		
CHEST		
LEFT ARM		
RIGHT ARM		
WAIST		
HIPS		
LEFT THIGH		
RIGHT THIGH		
LEFT CALF		
RIGHT CALF		
WEIGHT		
NOTES		

BODY MEASUREMENTS TRACKER

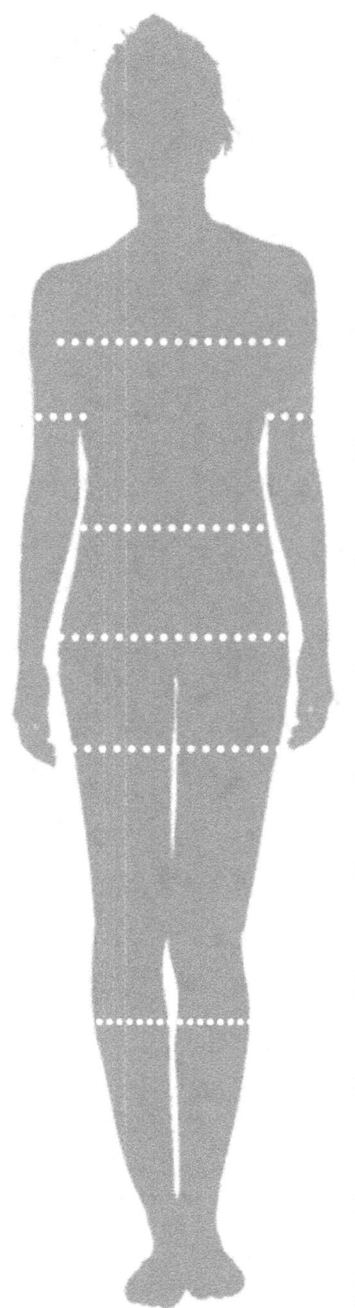

	BEFORE	AFTER
DATE		
CHEST		
LEFT ARM		
RIGHT ARM		
WAIST		
HIPS		
LEFT THIGH		
RIGHT THIGH		
LEFT CALF		
RIGHT CALF		
WEIGHT		
NOTES		

BODY MEASUREMENTS TRACKER

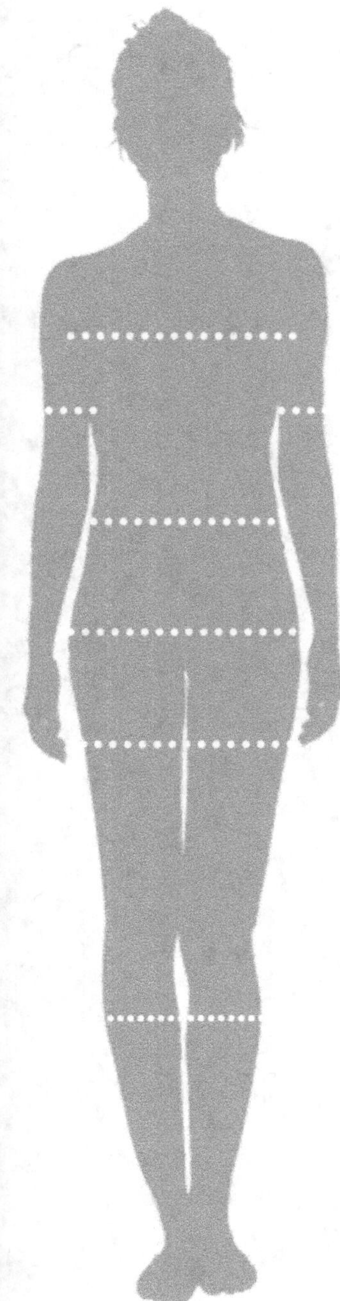

	BEFORE	AFTER
DATE		
CHEST		
LEFT ARM		
RIGHT ARM		
WAIST		
HIPS		
LEFT THIGH		
RIGHT THIGH		
LEFT CALF		
RIGHT CALF		
WEIGHT		
NOTES		

BODY MEASUREMENTS TRACKER

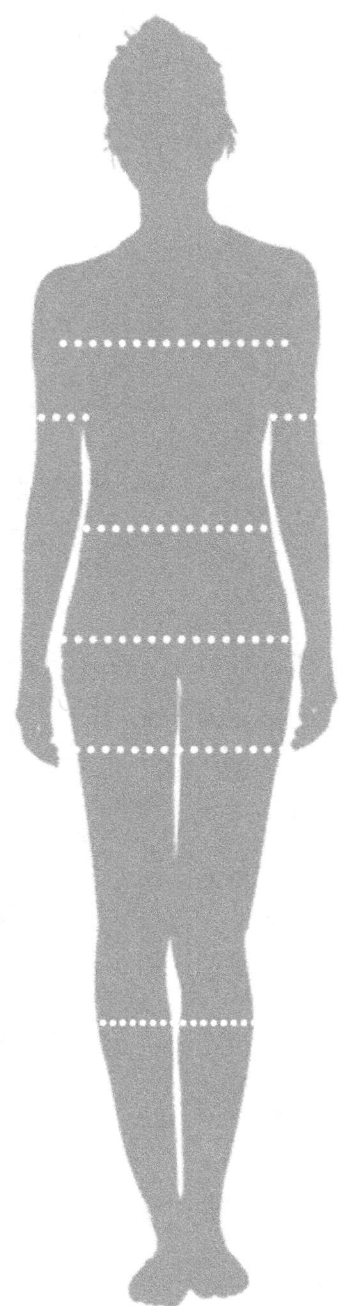

	BEFORE	AFTER
DATE		
CHEST		
LEFT ARM		
RIGHT ARM		
WAIST		
HIPS		
LEFT THIGH		
RIGHT THIGH		
LEFT CALF		
RIGHT CALF		
WEIGHT		
NOTES		

BODY MEASUREMENTS TRACKER

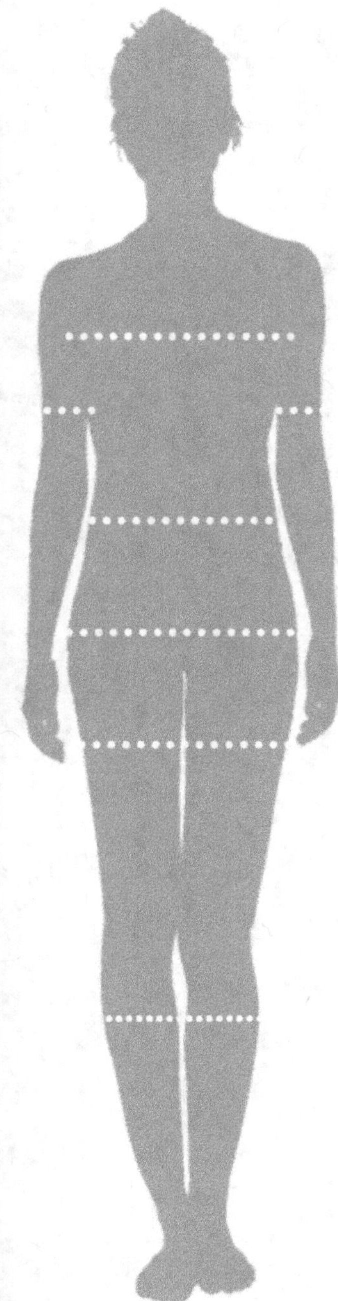

	BEFORE	AFTER
DATE		
CHEST		
LEFT ARM		
RIGHT ARM		
WAIST		
HIPS		
LEFT THIGH		
RIGHT THIGH		
LEFT CALF		
RIGHT CALF		
WEIGHT		
NOTES		

BODY MEASUREMENTS TRACKER

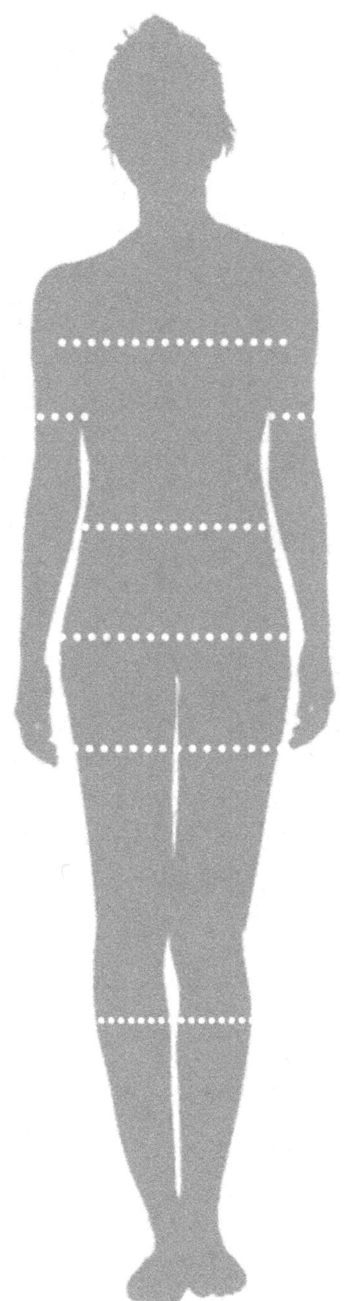

	BEFORE	AFTER
DATE		
CHEST		
LEFT ARM		
RIGHT ARM		
WAIST		
HIPS		
LEFT THIGH		
RIGHT THIGH		
LEFT CALF		
RIGHT CALF		
WEIGHT		
NOTES		

BODY MEASUREMENTS TRACKER

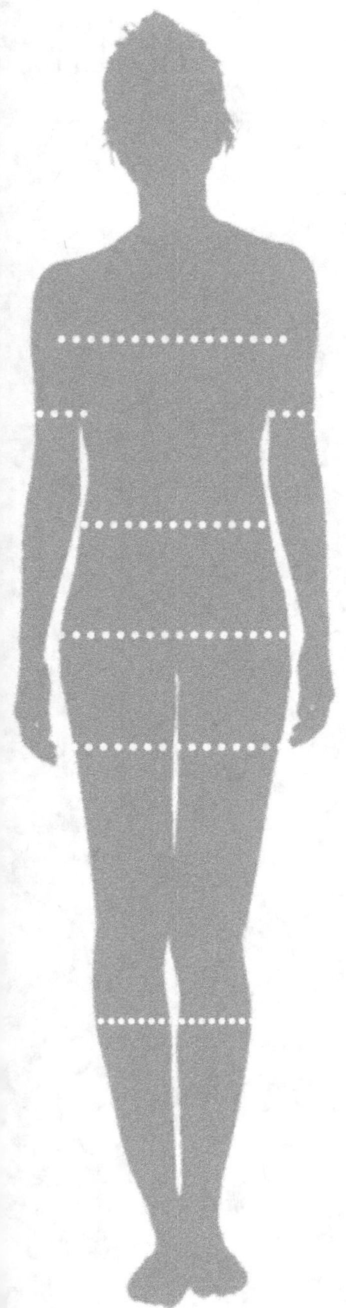

	BEFORE	AFTER
DATE		
CHEST		
LEFT ARM		
RIGHT ARM		
WAIST		
HIPS		
LEFT THIGH		
RIGHT THIGH		
LEFT CALF		
RIGHT CALF		
WEIGHT		
NOTES		

BODY MEASUREMENTS TRACKER

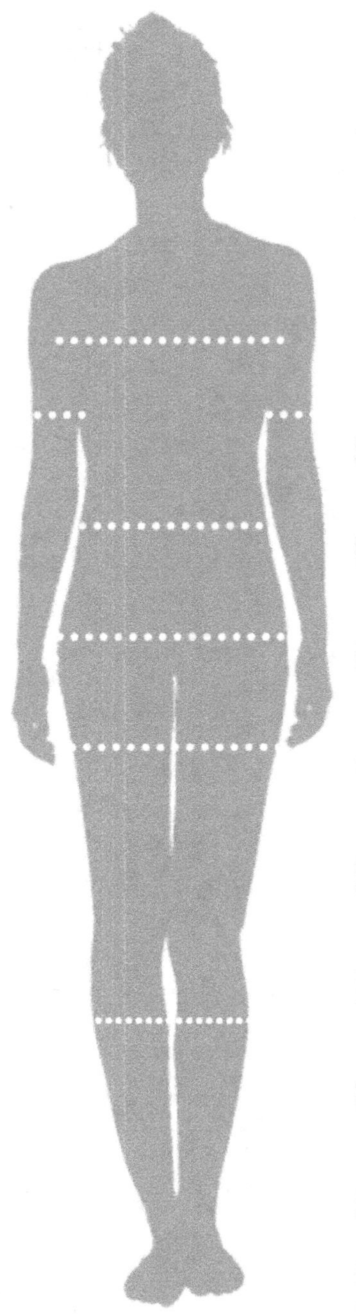

	BEFORE	AFTER
DATE		
CHEST		
LEFT ARM		
RIGHT ARM		
WAIST		
HIPS		
LEFT THIGH		
RIGHT THIGH		
LEFT CALF		
RIGHT CALF		
WEIGHT		
NOTES		

BODY MEASUREMENTS TRACKER

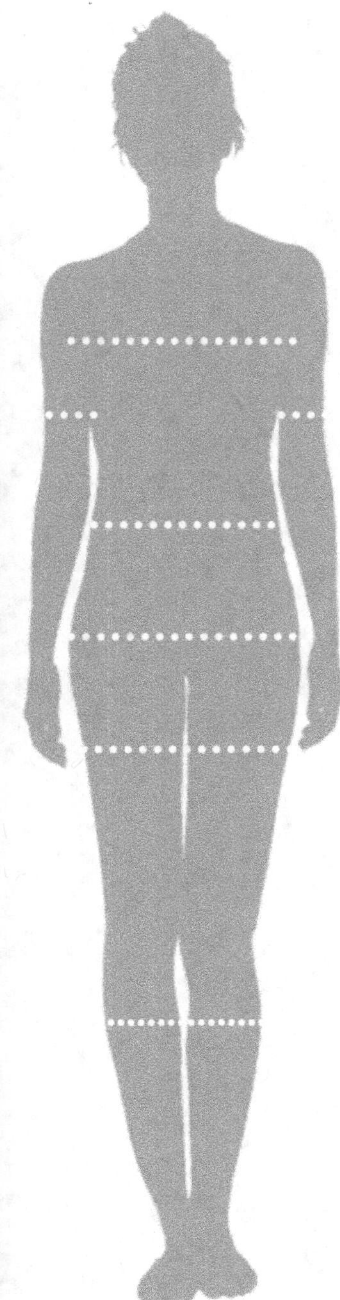

	BEFORE	AFTER
DATE		
CHEST		
LEFT ARM		
RIGHT ARM		
WAIST		
HIPS		
LEFT THIGH		
RIGHT THIGH		
LEFT CALF		
RIGHT CALF		
WEIGHT		
NOTES		

BODY MEASUREMENTS TRACKER

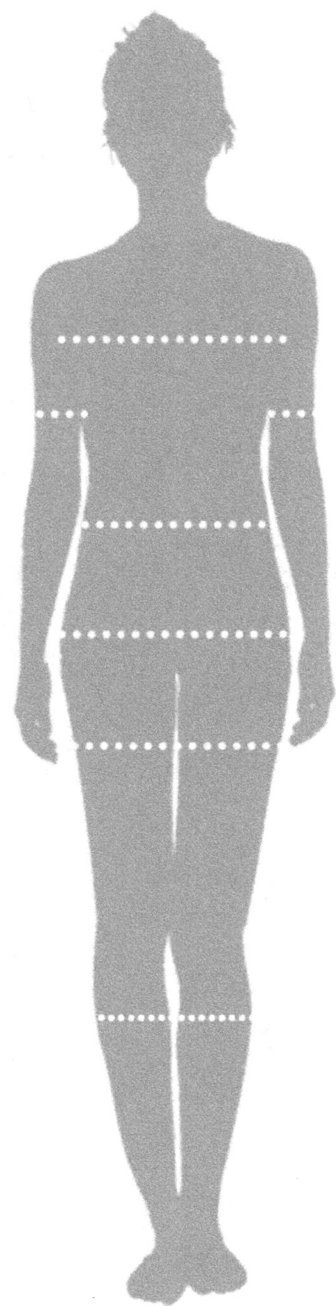

	BEFORE	AFTER
DATE		
CHEST		
LEFT ARM		
RIGHT ARM		
WAIST		
HIPS		
LEFT THIGH		
RIGHT THIGH		
LEFT CALF		
RIGHT CALF		
WEIGHT		
NOTES		

BODY MEASUREMENTS TRACKER

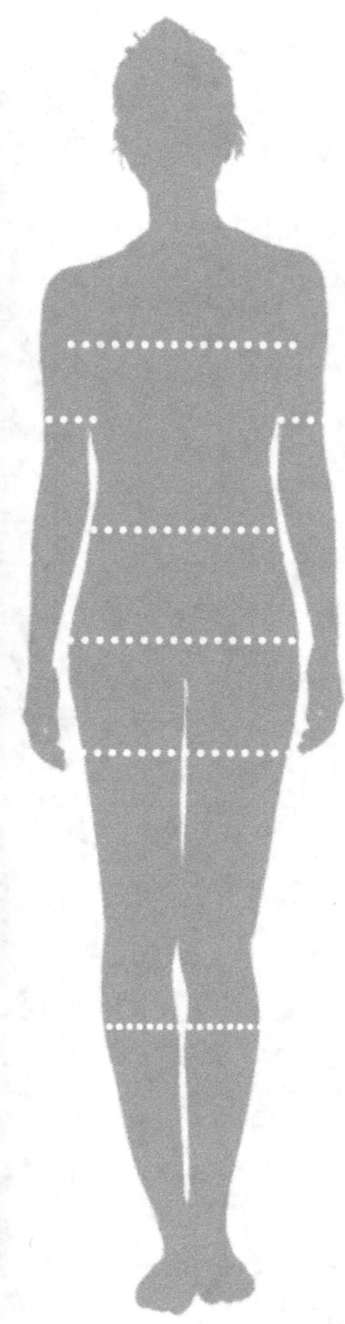

	BEFORE	AFTER
DATE		
CHEST		
LEFT ARM		
RIGHT ARM		
WAIST		
HIPS		
LEFT THIGH		
RIGHT THIGH		
LEFT CALF		
RIGHT CALF		
WEIGHT		
NOTES		

BODY MEASUREMENTS TRACKER

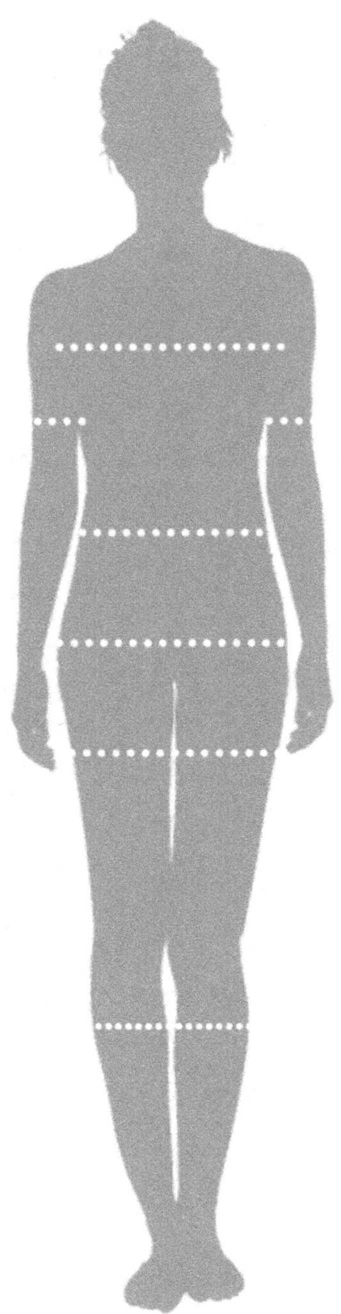

	BEFORE	AFTER
DATE		
CHEST		
LEFT ARM		
RIGHT ARM		
WAIST		
HIPS		
LEFT THIGH		
RIGHT THIGH		
LEFT CALF		
RIGHT CALF		
WEIGHT		
NOTES		

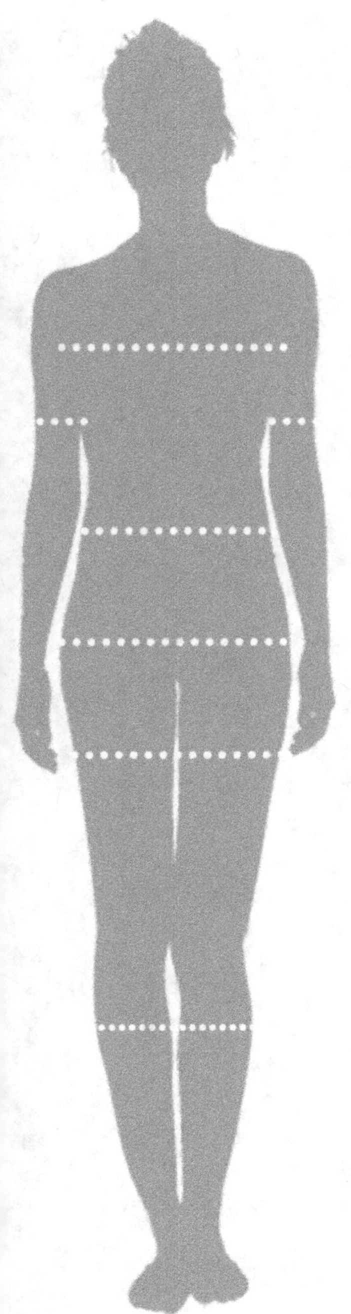

BODY MEASUREMENTS TRACKER

	BEFORE	AFTER
DATE		
CHEST		
LEFT ARM		
RIGHT ARM		
WAIST		
HIPS		
LEFT THIGH		
RIGHT THIGH		
LEFT CALF		
RIGHT CALF		
WEIGHT		
NOTES		

BODY MEASUREMENTS TRACKER

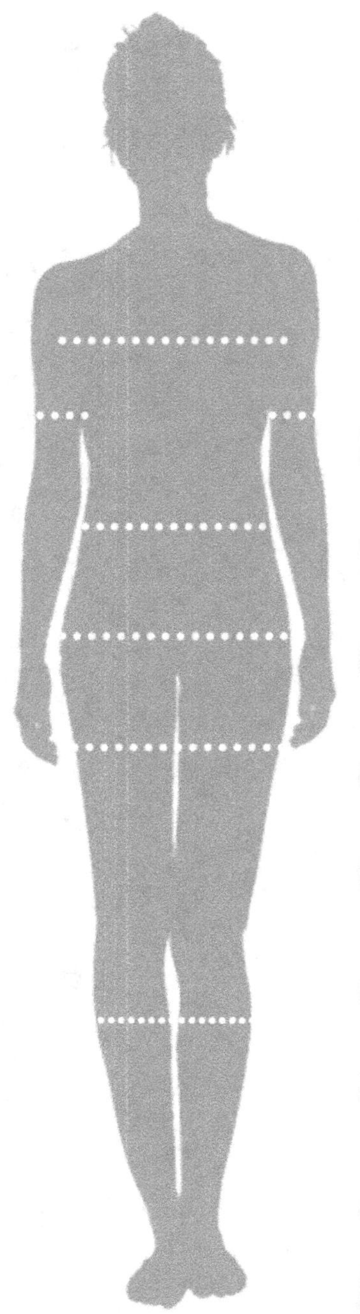

	BEFORE	AFTER
DATE		
CHEST		
LEFT ARM		
RIGHT ARM		
WAIST		
HIPS		
LEFT THIGH		
RIGHT THIGH		
LEFT CALF		
RIGHT CALF		
WEIGHT		
NOTES		

BODY MEASUREMENTS TRACKER

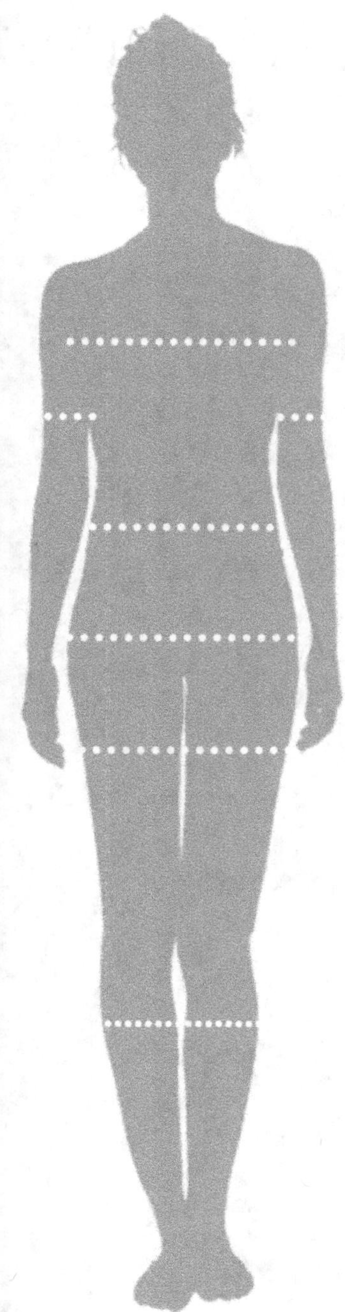

	BEFORE	AFTER
DATE		
CHEST		
LEFT ARM		
RIGHT ARM		
WAIST		
HIPS		
LEFT THIGH		
RIGHT THIGH		
LEFT CALF		
RIGHT CALF		
WEIGHT		
NOTES		

BODY MEASUREMENTS TRACKER

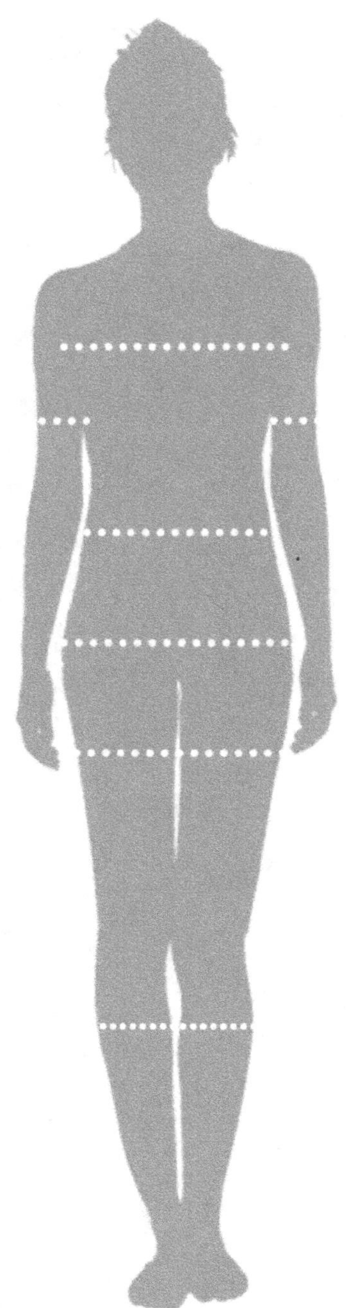

	BEFORE	AFTER
DATE		
CHEST		
LEFT ARM		
RIGHT ARM		
WAIST		
HIPS		
LEFT THIGH		
RIGHT THIGH		
LEFT CALF		
RIGHT CALF		
WEIGHT		
NOTES		

BODY MEASUREMENTS TRACKER

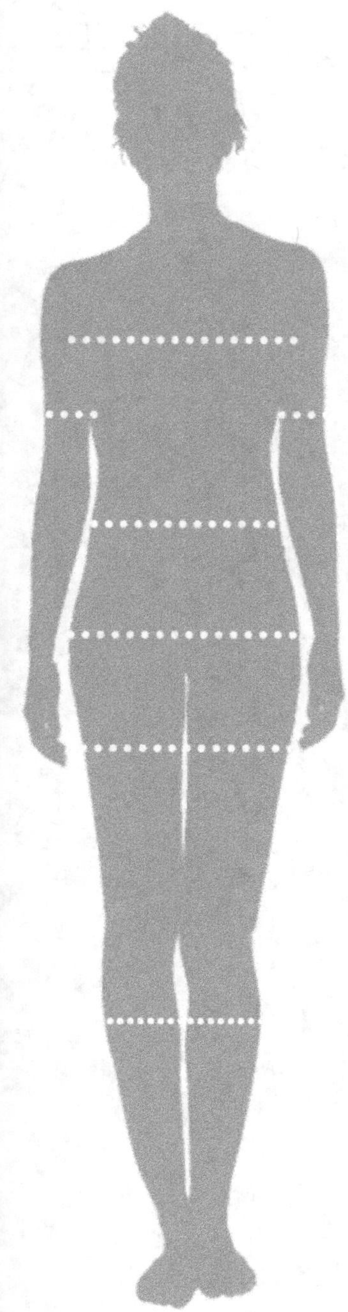

BEFORE

DATE

CHEST

LEFT ARM

RIGHT ARM

WAIST

HIPS

LEFT THIGH

RIGHT THIGH

LEFT CALF

RIGHT CALF

WEIGHT

NOTES

AFTER

DATE

CHEST

LEFT ARM

RIGHT ARM

WAIST

HIPS

LEFT THIGH

RIGHT THIGH

LEFT CALF

RIGHT CALF

WEIGHT

BODY MEASUREMENTS TRACKER

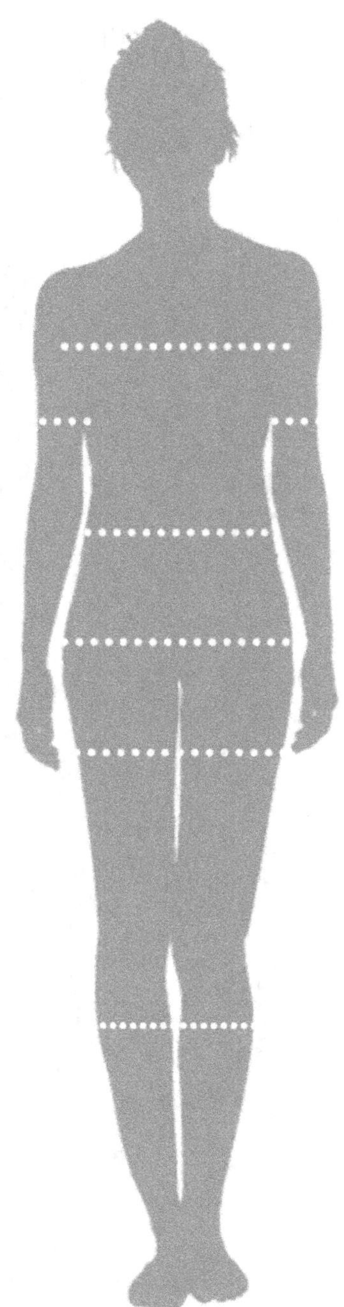

	BEFORE	AFTER
DATE		
CHEST		
LEFT ARM		
RIGHT ARM		
WAIST		
HIPS		
LEFT THIGH		
RIGHT THIGH		
LEFT CALF		
RIGHT CALF		
WEIGHT		
NOTES		

BODY MEASUREMENTS TRACKER

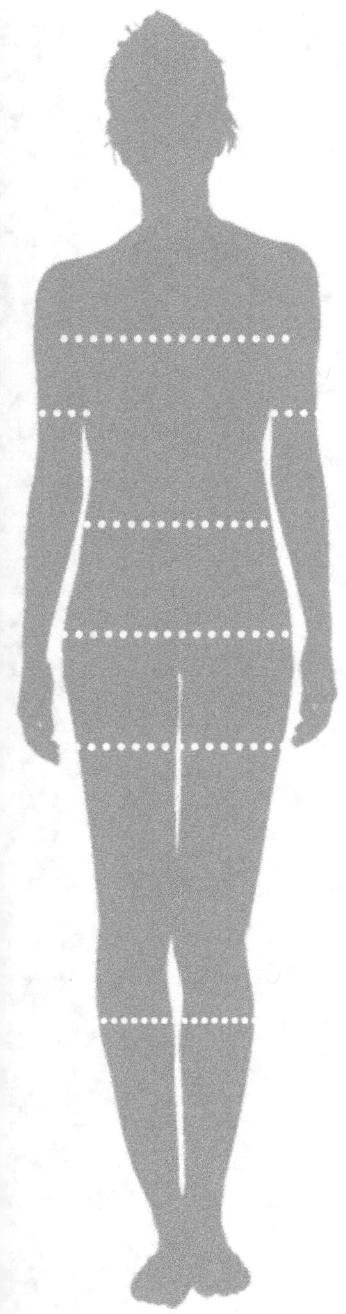

	BEFORE	AFTER
DATE		
CHEST		
LEFT ARM		
RIGHT ARM		
WAIST		
HIPS		
LEFT THIGH		
RIGHT THIGH		
LEFT CALF		
RIGHT CALF		
WEIGHT		
NOTES		

BODY MEASUREMENTS TRACKER

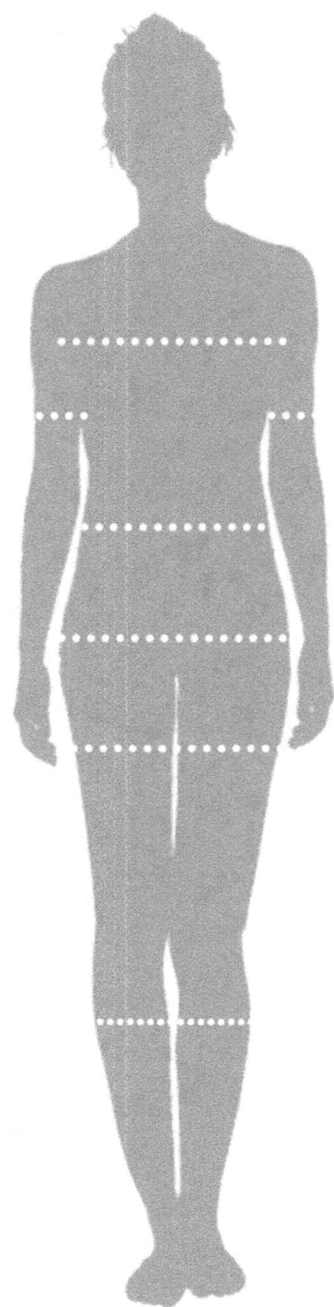

	BEFORE	AFTER
DATE		
CHEST		
LEFT ARM		
RIGHT ARM		
WAIST		
HIPS		
LEFT THIGH		
RIGHT THIGH		
LEFT CALF		
RIGHT CALF		
WEIGHT		
NOTES		

BODY MEASUREMENTS TRACKER

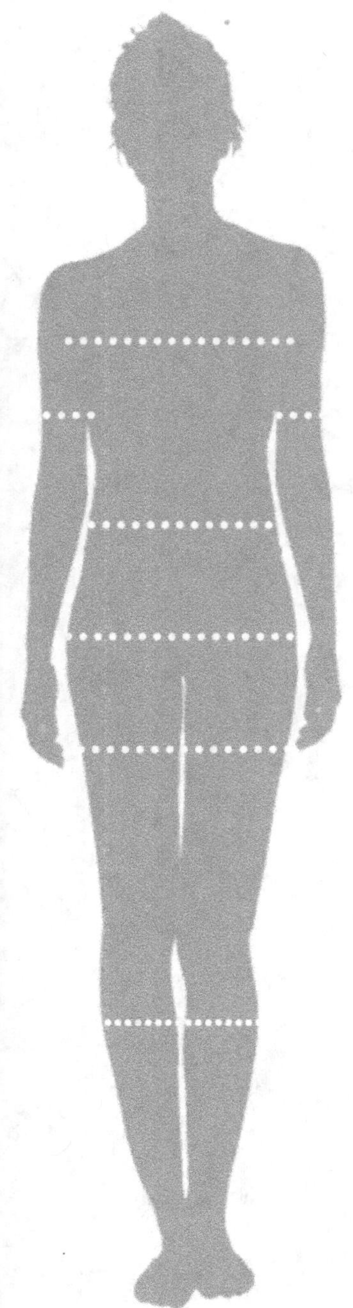

	BEFORE	AFTER
DATE		
CHEST		
LEFT ARM		
RIGHT ARM		
WAIST		
HIPS		
LEFT THIGH		
RIGHT THIGH		
LEFT CALF		
RIGHT CALF		
WEIGHT		
NOTES		

BODY MEASUREMENTS TRACKER

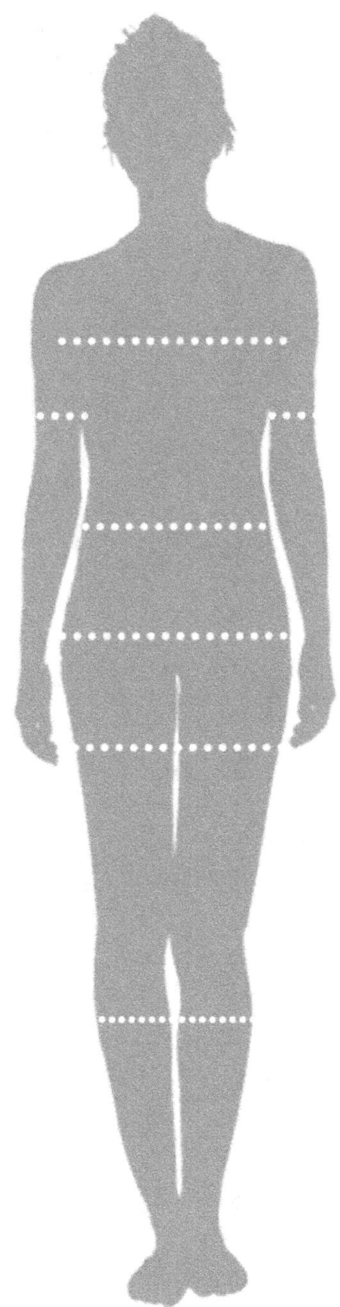

	BEFORE	AFTER
DATE		
CHEST		
LEFT ARM		
RIGHT ARM		
WAIST		
HIPS		
LEFT THIGH		
RIGHT THIGH		
LEFT CALF		
RIGHT CALF		
WEIGHT		
NOTES		

BODY MEASUREMENTS TRACKER

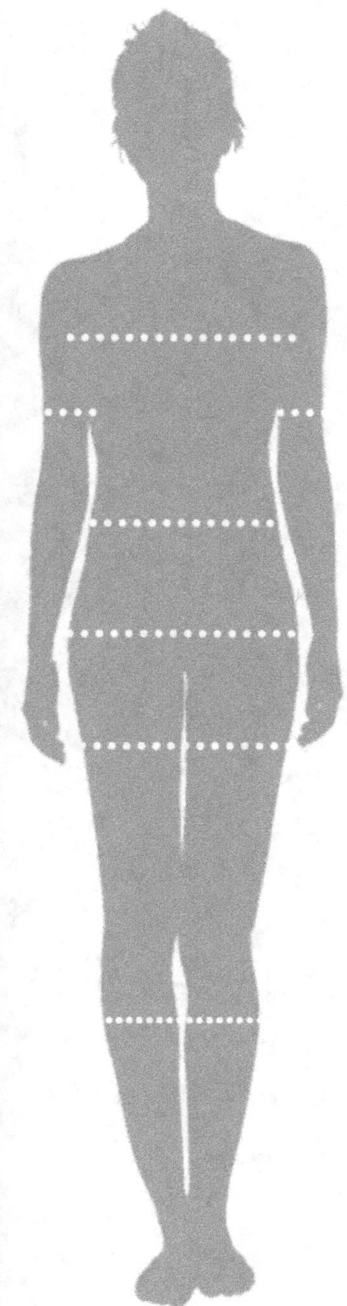

	BEFORE	AFTER
DATE		
CHEST		
LEFT ARM		
RIGHT ARM		
WAIST		
HIPS		
LEFT THIGH		
RIGHT THIGH		
LEFT CALF		
RIGHT CALF		
WEIGHT		
NOTES		

BODY MEASUREMENTS TRACKER

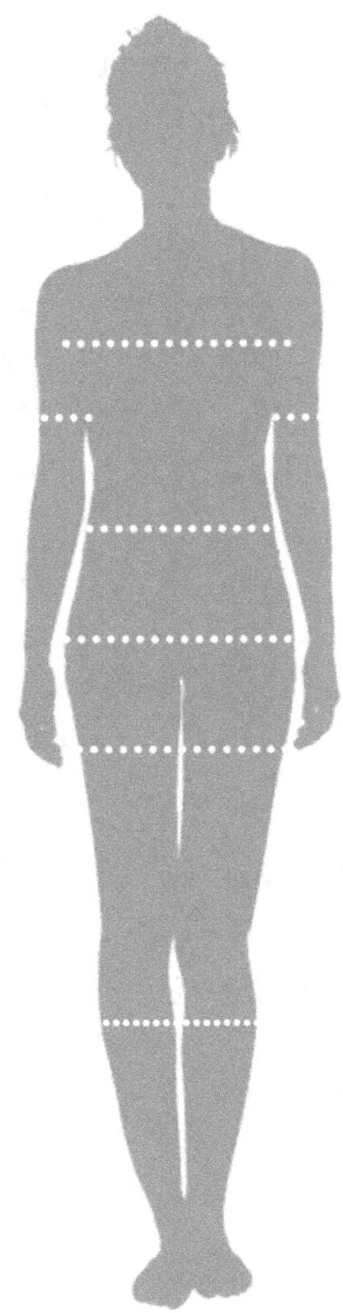

	BEFORE	AFTER
DATE		
CHEST		
LEFT ARM		
RIGHT ARM		
WAIST		
HIPS		
LEFT THIGH		
RIGHT THIGH		
LEFT CALF		
RIGHT CALF		
WEIGHT		
NOTES		

BODY MEASUREMENTS TRACKER

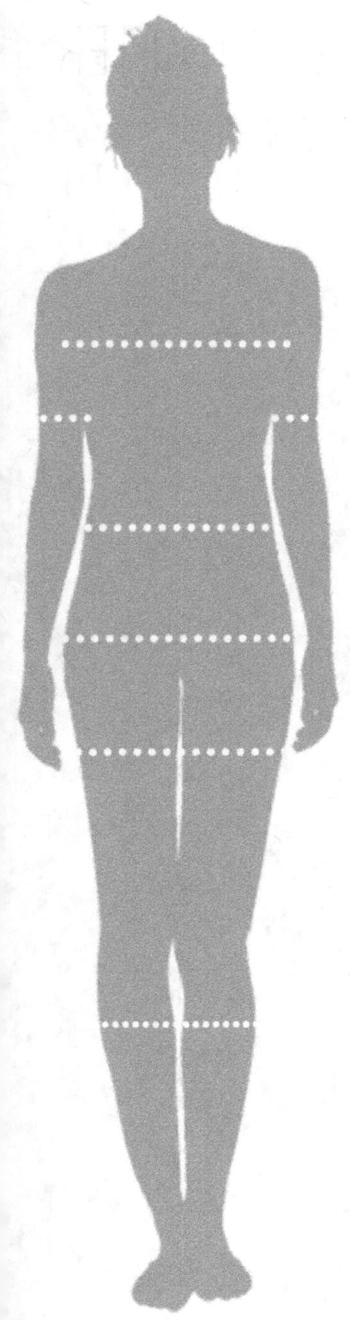

	BEFORE	AFTER
DATE		
CHEST		
LEFT ARM		
RIGHT ARM		
WAIST		
HIPS		
LEFT THIGH		
RIGHT THIGH		
LEFT CALF		
RIGHT CALF		
WEIGHT		
NOTES		

BODY MEASUREMENTS TRACKER

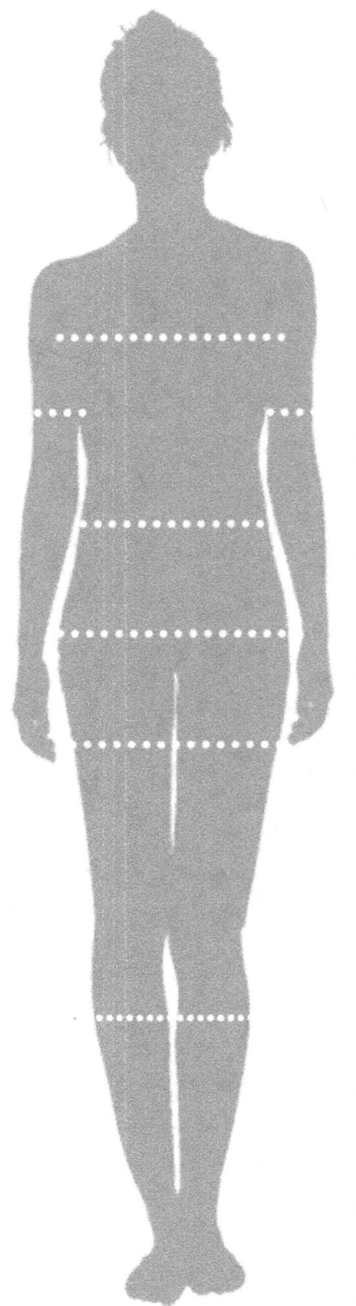

	BEFORE	AFTER
DATE		
CHEST		
LEFT ARM		
RIGHT ARM		
WAIST		
HIPS		
LEFT THIGH		
RIGHT THIGH		
LEFT CALF		
RIGHT CALF		
WEIGHT		
NOTES		

BODY MEASUREMENTS TRACKER

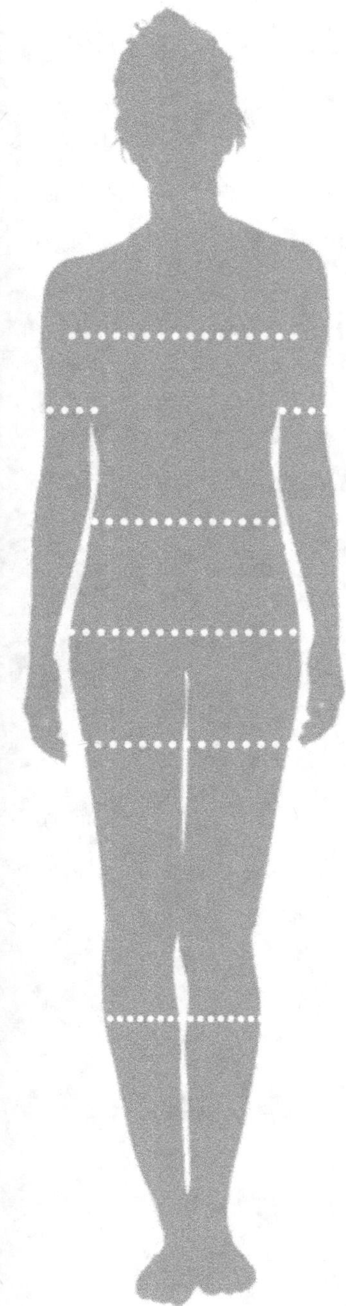

	BEFORE	AFTER
DATE		
CHEST		
LEFT ARM		
RIGHT ARM		
WAIST		
HIPS		
LEFT THIGH		
RIGHT THIGH		
LEFT CALF		
RIGHT CALF		
WEIGHT		
NOTES		

BODY MEASUREMENTS TRACKER

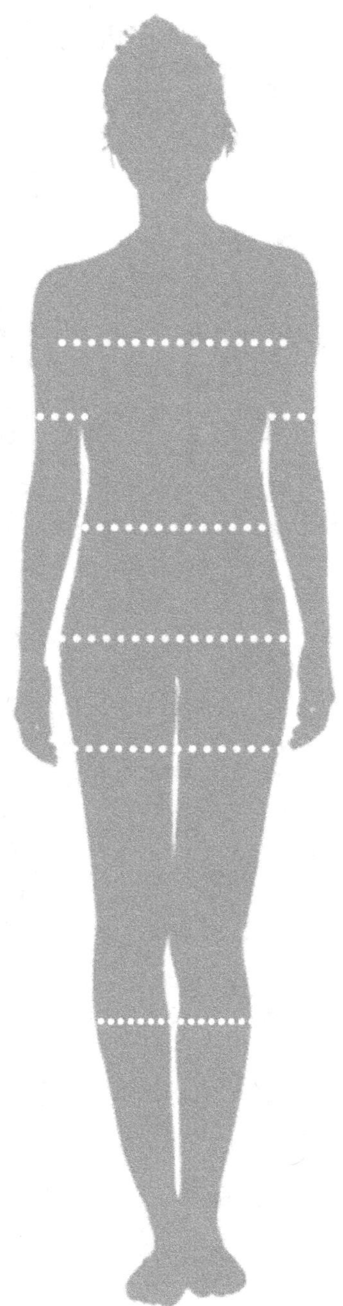

BEFORE

DATE

CHEST

LEFT ARM

RIGHT ARM

WAIST

HIPS

LEFT THIGH

RIGHT THIGH

LEFT CALF

RIGHT CALF

WEIGHT

NOTES

AFTER

DATE

CHEST

LEFT ARM

RIGHT ARM

WAIST

HIPS

LEFT THIGH

RIGHT THIGH

LEFT CALF

RIGHT CALF

WEIGHT

BODY MEASUREMENTS TRACKER

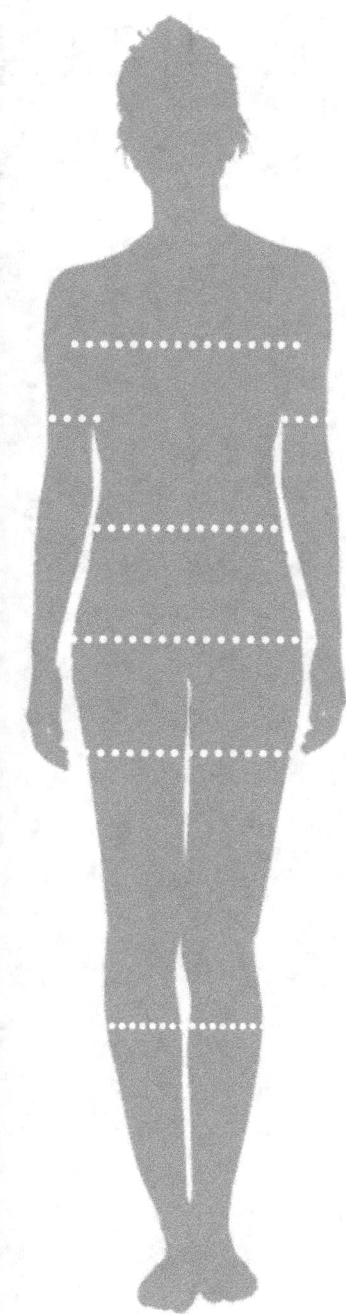

BEFORE

DATE

CHEST

LEFT ARM

RIGHT ARM

WAIST

HIPS

LEFT THIGH

RIGHT THIGH

LEFT CALF

RIGHT CALF

WEIGHT

NOTES

AFTER

DATE

CHEST

LEFT ARM

RIGHT ARM

WAIST

HIPS

LEFT THIGH

RIGHT THIGH

LEFT CALF

RIGHT CALF

WEIGHT

BODY MEASUREMENTS TRACKER

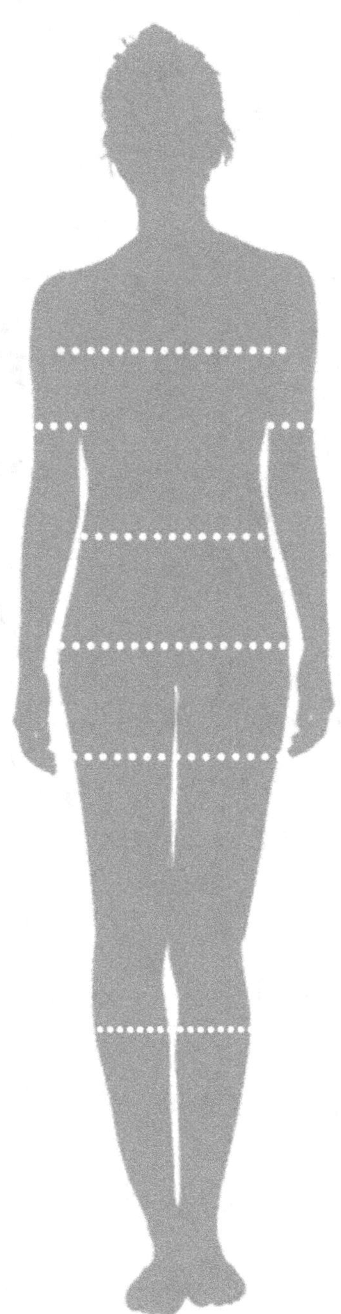

	BEFORE	AFTER
DATE		
CHEST		
LEFT ARM		
RIGHT ARM		
WAIST		
HIPS		
LEFT THIGH		
RIGHT THIGH		
LEFT CALF		
RIGHT CALF		
WEIGHT		
NOTES